Storytelling Online

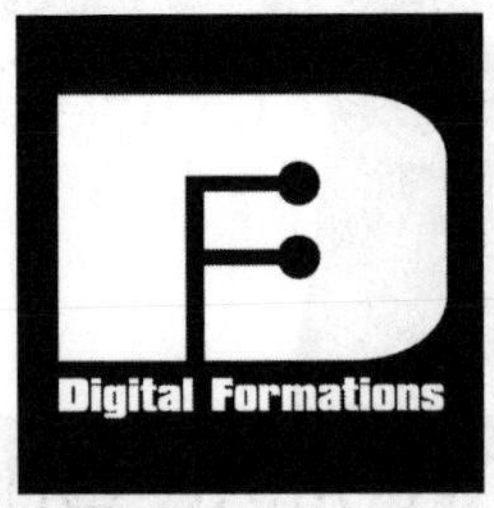

Steve Jones
General Editor

Vol. 29

PETER LANG
New York • Washington, D.C./Baltimore • Bern
Frankfurt am Main • Berlin • Brussels • Vienna • Oxford

SHANI ORGAD

Storytelling Online

Talking Breast Cancer on the Internet

PETER LANG
New York • Washington, D.C./Baltimore • Bern
Frankfurt am Main • Berlin • Brussels • Vienna • Oxford

Library of Congress Cataloging-in-Publication Data

Orgad, Shani.
Storytelling online: talking breast cancer on the Internet / Shani Orgad.
p. cm. — (Digital formations; v. 29)
Includes bibliographical references and index.
1. Breast—Cancer—Computer network resources.
2. Breast—Cancer—Social aspects. 3. Internet—Social aspects.
4. Internet in medicine. I. Title. II. Series.
RC280.B80745 362.196'99449—dc22 2004027917
ISBN 0-8204-7629-3
ISSN 1526-3169

Bibliographic information published by **Die Deutsche Bibliothek**.
Die Deutsche Bibliothek lists this publication in the "Deutsche Nationalbibliografie"; detailed bibliographic data is available on the Internet at http://dnb.ddb.de/.

Cover design by Joni Holst
Cover image: *the rules*, by Jennifer Davis (jenniferdavisart.com)

The paper in this book meets the guidelines for permanence and durability of the Committee on Production Guidelines for Book Longevity of the Council of Library Resources.

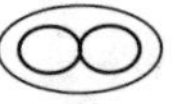

275 Seventh Avenue, 28th Floor, New York, NY 10001
www.peterlangusa.com

Printed in the United States of America

Disclaimer

> [T]he task of transforming a living person into a character ties the hand of the writer. This happens because such a task, even when it is undertaken with the best intentions and deals with a respected and loved person, verges on the violation of privacy and is never painless for the subject.
>
> Primo Levi
> *Moments of Reprieve* (1979)

I have made every possible effort to cause as little harm as possible to all the individuals whose online and offline stories I have incorporated into my account. Nevertheless, despite my best efforts, I might still have hurt somebody's feelings. If this is the case, I invite the reader to contact me at s.s.orgad@lse.ac.uk

Contents

Figures

Acronyms

ASCC	American Society for Cancer Control
BCANS	Breast Cancer Action Nova Scotia
CA	Conversation Analysis
CMC	Computer Mediated Communication
IRC	Internet Relay Chat
NHS	National Health Service

Acknowledgments

The writing of this book has been a process of discovery, where many precious people have been with me or have just been there for me when I needed support.

The book could have never been written without the generous participation of many dear women, and two men, whom I met and interviewed online and offline. My deepest gratitude goes to all those who were willing to tell me their personal stories of using the Internet in relation to their illness or that of their dearly loved. This book acknowledges not just those whose stories I have been able to quote, but also the many others that I came across online and offline, and who were key to my exploration.

The book is based on my doctoral research, and I am thankful to my supervisor, Roger Silverstone, who guided me in this project, and always urged me to keep rethinking and discovering new angles and aspects. I'm also very grateful to Richard Sennett, who gave me counsel, motivation and faith, to imagine and explore. Special thanks go to Robin Mansell and Terhi Rantanen, who provided constructive advice as well as constant encouragement. I owe thanks also to many other friends and colleagues at the LSE who provided invaluable support. Thanks to Terry Halsey for permission to use figures from the "Shared Experience" website, and to Jennifer Davis for permission to reprint her artwork on the book cover.

Many thanks go to Corinne Vella, who escorted this long process from its early stages, as a professional copyeditor and a dear friend. My gratitude goes also to Cynthia Little, who scrutinized every page of this book, with tremendous care and professionalism.

I acknowledge with great appreciation the funding of my Ph.D. studies by the Doctoral Scholarship of Tel Aviv University, the Anglo Jewish Association, and the LSE for their generous support. The pursuance of this project would have been impossible without these bodies' assistance.

Finally, my deepest debt is to my family. My mother, Atalya Wolf, has always been there for me with her unfailing love. Very special thanks go to Kobi Wolf, Nechemya Orgad, Itamar and Ifat Orgad, Tanya and Noam Gilboa-Greenberg, Dalia Habshush, Barbara and Shmuel Jashinski and Shai Aran. My greatest appreciation to my dearest friend and beloved husband, Amnon Aran. All the possible synonyms for "loving" and "caring" would not adequately capture what he has been for me in this challenging process.

Last but not least, special thanks to all the wonderful people in Peter Lang with whom it has been a great pleasure to work: Steve Jones, the series' editor, Damon Zucca, Bernadette Shade and the many others involved in the making of this book.

CHAPTER 1

Introduction: The Story of This Book

> The art of storytelling is coming to an end.
>
> Walter Benjamin
> *The Storyteller, Illuminations* (1970)

> All sorrows can be borne if you put them into a story or tell a story about them.
>
> Isak Dinesen, cited in Hannah Arendt
> *The Human Condition* (1958)

This book is a sociological study of breast cancer patients' participation in Internet spaces. While this may seem a quite specific and even distinctive context to study, a broader intellectual question underlies the inquiry: the social significance of the Internet in people's lives. Sweeping claims are constantly made regarding the significance or insignificance of this communicative technology, but the actual processes of communication in which people engage online, and the consequences for their lives, are little understood as yet. So when I chose this particular context my goal was to inquire into the processes, practices and forms that are involved in participants' online communication, and to try to ascertain to what extent computer mediated communication (CMC) is a socially meaningful activity. These are obviously huge questions, and there are many possible ways to address them empirically. I chose to focus on a particular empirical context, namely, the online communication of breast cancer patients. You might justifiably ask yourself why.

In recent years breast cancer online spaces have proliferated, especially those oriented to patient resources (Fogel, Albert, Schnabel, Ditkoff and Neugut, 2002; Pitts, 2004; Sharf, 1997). The abundance of various kinds of online communication related to breast cancer seems especially salient given the high prevalence of breast cancer and its centrality in contemporary society. Furthermore, the profusion of diverse activities, forums and forms of patients' communication on the Internet contrasts starkly with the silence and lack of visibility in the public arena that has characterized the illness until recently. For many decades women who suffered with breast cancer had no infrastructure to communicate the disease (Leopold, 1999). Today the situation is significantly different. The online space constitutes a central space in the widening infrastructure for the communication of the illness in contemporary society, particularly by the patients themselves. For these reasons the online communication of breast cancer patients seemed a particularly suitable context to examine the broader question of the social significance of the Internet in people's lives.

There is another, more personal reason behind my decision to take breast cancer patients' online communication as the core topic for this study. More than forty-five years ago my grandmother was diagnosed with breast cancer. At the time of her diagnosis and throughout the following years, very few people knew about her illness. Those who did, knew very little. The experience of her illness was never discussed. The silence that surrounded it contrasts starkly with what the contemporary online space seems to offer: a vibrant and active communicative space, where women share their experience and exchange it with each other in various forms and ways. On any of the major search engines, the key words "breast cancer" retrieve hundreds of related websites full of information on the disease, as well as patients' forums such as message boards, mailing lists, personal columns, journals, diaries and chats. So my grandmother's experience, and its contrast with what women may experience today, is the backdrop to my interest in exploring contemporary online environments of breast cancer patients.

I began my inquiry with two key research questions: what kinds of processes, practices, structures and forms are involved in the online experience of women who suffer from breast cancer and what makes these online spaces attractive and thereby arguably meaningful to their participants. To date, the search for information is the most common explanation. Patients' online engagement in the context of health, and particularly that of chronic illness such as breast cancer, was regarded primarily and often exclusively as an act of seeking, sharing and appropriating information (e.g., Eastin, 2001; Pew Internet & American Life, 2003). The claim for the significance of these activities and, by association, of the online environments in which patients engage, lies in the idea that "information is power." The argument goes that since information is empowering (a view that has been too often taken uncritically), in providing patients with cheap, direct and easy access to a variety of informative sites and resources, the Internet can potentially empower patients. Within this premise, studies have often been concerned with aspects of the verifiability, credibility, trustworthiness and accuracy of the information on these sites, the purpose being to ascertain the empowering potential of different health-related online spaces.

It should be said, however, that there are studies of individuals' online communication (albeit fewer regarding patients) that do not see information as the key to explaining the social significance of CMC. Researchers working on this premise focus on exploring interpersonal opportunities facilitated by CMC. They perceive the significance of the Internet and CMC primarily for processes of identity construction and self-presentation (e.g., Turkle, 1996; Walker, 2000; Wynn and Katz, 1997), development and maintenance of relationships (e.g., Baker, 2002; Baym, 2000) and expression of emotions (e.g., Preece and Ghozati, 2001; Rice and Love, 1987).

Their accounts shed light on the question of the social significance of online communication for breast cancer patients. However, they do not account for something else that seems to be going on. Participants in breast cancer sites engage in a communicative process that cannot be fully understood by existing models, and that has not been studied in depth so far. This process, I suggest, can be described as storytelling.

Storytelling Online as a Socially Meaningful Activity

Storytelling refers to the process by which participants in online spaces configure their experience (or at least struggle to do so) into a story. Perhaps the most explicit manifestation of this process can be seen on patients' personal home pages where they talk about their illness experience in a narrated form. For example:

> **My Story**
>
> In 1985, at the age of 36 when I was first diagnosed with breast cancer, the perception of this disease was quite different. There was no breast cancer awareness, there was not an understanding of the disease, no support systems and definitely not many options available. There were however many misconceptions. (A breast cancer personal online journal)

As in the example above, participants often refer to the texts they publish online as their "story," whether they are in the form of a personal diary or a text on a message board, on a mailing list or in some other space. Yet the process of storytelling is much more complex than its manifestation in the "final product" of a story published online. It involves myriad practices and processes that are part of the participants' struggle to produce a story, to construct a framework to organize their experience into a coherent text that can be communicated back to themselves, and to others. These practices and processes are at the heart of this book.

The key argument in this book is that the online experience furnishes breast cancer patients with, among other things, a means and a space to configure their experience into a story. Storytelling online is a potentially meaningful activity because it constitutes a way in which patients maintain and develop agency. That is, it is a process that enables patients to hold on to a sense of themselves as agents who have control, however little, over their lives. This process appears particularly pertinent in light of the recognition of cancer as a disturbance to everyday life. Patients' engagement in online spaces is understood as part of their attempt to regain the fundamentals disturbed by cancer (a theoretical assertion I develop in Chapter 3). By exploring patients' engagement in storytelling in their online experience, my aim is to shed light on the significance of CMC for their capacity to cope with their illness.

Needless to say, patients engage in several types of communicative processes online. As shown by recent studies, and corroborated by the patients' accounts in this research, in going online, different patients do different things, at different stages in their illness, and for different purposes. They seek, appropriate and exchange information (e.g., Eastin, 2001; McLellan, 1997; Pew Internet & American Life, 2003), share experience and emotions (e.g., Preece and Ghozati, 2001; Sharf, 1997), ask questions, lurk (as I discuss in Chapter 5) and tell stories (e.g., Eley, 2003; Hardey, 2002). All of these activities and processes are salient, as are the studies that explore them. However, the focus of this study is on the latter, that is, storytelling. Significantly, this book does not assert storytelling to be an overarching way to understand participants' online communication, nor is it a prescriptive model of what patients do online. What this book tries to do is to highlight storytelling as one possible way to explain participants' online experience. In short, it develops storytelling as a model for understanding online communication as a socially meaningful activity.

Consequently, the focus of the book is not the storytellers, that is, the online participants, but rather the work of making and telling their stories. This differs from studies on Internet use, whose concern is to characterize the population of Internet users (e.g., Anderson and Tracey, 2002; Hoffman, Novak and Schlosser, 2001; Nie and Erbring, 2000). This latter kind of study is particularly common in the research field of online health, where the aim is often to construct typologies of "health seekers" or "e-patients" and their online activities (e.g., Pew Internet & American Life, 2000, 2003). Put simply, this study is concerned with understanding the process of storytelling and its social significance, rather than identifying and characterizing the people who engage in this process.

The remainder of this introduction has three major objectives. The first is to contextualize the research empirically and methodologically. The empirical part introduces the reader to the landscape of patients' online communication of breast cancer. This overview expands on the reasons I chose this particular context to examine the broader question of the social significance of online communication, and of storytelling in particular. I also describe the study I conducted and its key stages. This background is necessary for the reader to understand how I obtained and analyzed the data used throughout the book. Second, I discuss the key theoretical areas within which and against which I locate my study. The theoretical discussion that follows the empirical and methodological account is a critical overview of current research on health online, particularly patients' online communication and even more particularly the work done on patients' online communication in relation to breast cancer. It also discusses the few studies that include storytelling and narrative in their exploration of CMC, highlighting their strengths and weaknesses. However, given their neglect or scant attention to storytelling, the theoretical foundations for this book are to be found largely beyond the literature in this field. These theoretical foundations are discussed in depth in Chapter 2, and employed throughout the book. The last part of the theoretical discussion is a critique of the omission of ideas on storytelling and narrative in the current debate on the Internet and CMC. I try to explain this gap in the literature, stressing the need to pay attention to storytelling as a useful model for understanding participants' online communication as a socially significant experience. Finally, the last part of this chapter presents the structure of the book.

Empirical and Methodological Context: The Landscape of Breast Cancer Patients' Online Communication

Online, breast cancer is a highly communicated topic. There are hundreds of websites focusing on different aspects of the disease and its treatment. On other more generic websites that deal with areas such as cancer, chronic illness or health, breast cancer is often the most prominent topic, both quantitatively (the proportion of the website that it occupies) and qualitatively (for instance, in terms of its visibility and centrality in comparison to other topics). Significantly, in interactive spaces focused on chronic illness, particularly cancer, the most active forums are the ones that deal with breast cancer. For example, at the time of writing this chapter, in the "Shared Experience" website,[1] about a quarter (536) of all cancer patients' stories (2,260) were about breast cancer. In "The Cancer Survivors Network" of the American Cancer Society's discussion board,[2] more than 60% of the messages (16,943) regarding experience of cancer are related to breast cancer.

Of course, the prominence of the topic in online spaces is tied in with the material and social reality of the disease. The high prevalence of breast cancer is undoubtedly of concern: on average, one out of every eight women will suffer from breast cancer. In some countries the statistic is even higher. Breast cancer is a central experience in contemporary society, if only because everyone potentially knows someone who has or had the disease. When a chronic illness is so prominent in our everyday lives, its communication is highly consequential for its social reality.

Breast cancer-related websites commonly consist of informative textual features such as downloadable articles, medical research, statistics and glossaries of terms on aspects of a particular problem. There are also some informative visual features. For example, using Web camera technology, websites broadcast surgical operations to help patients prepare themselves for surgery. Most websites also have interactive forums such as peer group e-mails, message boards, discussion lists, newsletters, online personal diaries and text chat rooms. These forums facilitate patient–patient communication and patient–health professional communication. Many of the online forums have been founded by breast cancer patients and survivors who run websites to communicate the experience of their disease. Other websites are owned by commercial and nonprofit organizations and institutions.

Naturally, the majority of consistently active participants in those websites are women diagnosed with, or worried about, breast cancer. Breast cancer patients engage in various kinds of interaction including posting messages on message boards, sending e-mails to fellow sufferers, publishing their "journey with breast cancer" (as they often call their personal online diaries), discussing aspects of the illness in text chats, sending prayers on "praying message boards" to women undergoing risky stages in their treatment, and reading and responding to breast cancer mailing lists. The most notable participants in breast cancer-related online forums are patients who are going through the illness or those who have been through it. Other participants include friends and family, caregivers (other than family), members of medical organizations, medical workers and other related experts.

Researching the Online Communication of Breast Cancer

Getting Started

Over three and a half years, I followed different breast cancer online forums and activities. This included participating in breast cancer online message boards (albeit mostly by lurking), reading patients' personal online diaries, participating in breast cancer chats, browsing through informative sections in different breast cancer websites and maintaining long-term e-mail correspondence with patient-participants.

However, a neutral observer of breast cancer websites would find it difficult to completely make sense of what goes on there. Several questions come to mind. What motivates patients to go online in relation to their health condition in the first place? What causes them to actively participate, for instance, to disclose their experience on breast cancer message boards? Is participants' online engagement socially meaningful for them and, if so, in what sense? Merely observing messages and logs on breast cancer websites cannot provide satisfactory answers to these kinds of questions, because such texts are limited in their capacity to reveal the more complex stories behind these online appearances. For one thing, since the language of CMC is intended for people directly involved in online interactions, it tends to lose some of its sense and meaning when read by neutral observers (Reid, 1995, in Paccagnella, 1997).

Hence, although this "loose" participant observation of different online breast cancer spaces was absolutely necessary as a point of departure (and, as the research progressed, maintaining it on a continuous basis was significant), on its own it was obviously insufficient. There remained the need to obtain participants' constructions of their online experience. To do so, I first needed to gain access to the members of the group I wanted to study.

I wanted to focus only on women who suffer/suffered from breast cancer and experienced the Internet in the context of their illness. Focusing on this group meant excluding other groups, for example, men diagnosed with breast cancer (although the incidence of male breast cancer is rare when compared to the incidence of the disease in women), women with breast cancer who do not have access to the Internet and women who have access but who, for different reasons, do not go online in the context of their illness.

Gaining Access to Participants' Lives

Informants were initially recruited online. To obtain participants' constructions of their experience, I posted messages on online breast cancer message boards on health-related websites, expressing my interest in women who would agree to share with me their experience of using the Internet in the context of their illness. In addition, I directly e-mailed women who provided their e-mail addresses with the messages they posted on those boards. I repeated these procedures twice: first during December 1999–January 2000, and then during June–July 2001. In total I received eighty-three replies.

I believe that this good response rate is largely due to elements such as availability, degree of anonymity, high individual control of participation in the online interaction, and being comfortable with the medium. Arguably, similar factors had motivated these women to participate online in the context of their illness. In particular, many scholars suggest that the anonymity provided by electronic communication encourages the extent of self-disclosure and the degree of intimacy (Jones, 1998; Rheingold, 1994; Sharf, 1997). However, as I discuss later in this book, in the case of the online participants studied here, anonymity assumes a quite different meaning than the capacity to invent personas and disguise one's real identity.

All replies (with the exception of one account that arrived via snail mail) were sent to me by e-mail. I recontacted some of the women who initially replied and asked them to elaborate their accounts. Remarkably, most e-mails consisted of fairly detailed accounts of their online experience following their diagnosis with breast cancer.[3] Take, for example, the following e-mail account:

> I received my diagnosis (over the phone) on a Friday afternoon.
> **1** By 5 PM I was online, searching for all the info I could find.
>
> I am computer literate and comfortable surfing the web. It was
> comforting to know that I could look up whatever I wanted and
> do it in my PJs at 3 AM if I felt like it. I expected to find a lot on
> the web, what I did find and was not expecting was a HUGE
> group of breast cancer patients and survivors who became great
> sources of information and some became permanent friends. I
> started by typing BREAST CANCER into my search engine—and
> it just took off from there.
> There are medical links, chat rooms, message boards, you name
> it—you can find it! Tons of information you get from other
> women who have dealt with BC is different from what the doctor
> tells you. He tells you what the treatment should do, lists the
> possible sideeffects, recommends medications to combat the
> side effects, etc. The ladies have BEEN THERE, DONE THAT—
> they give you an honest accounting of how it happens, what it
> **2** feels like, what side effects are and how to handle them.
> Medical information I printed out and discussed with my doctor
> if I thought article was valid. I did NOT follow any medical regime without discussing with my doctors first. All the info from
> the BC ladies is their personal account of how they felt or dealt
> with BC and its treatments. Once in a while they would suggest
> something that I felt I had to ask my doctor about. (Example:
> BC warrior ladies tell you to shave your head at first sign of going bald—they say it is less itchy that way.) Nothing I had to
> confirm with my drs. Some recommended soy. Checked some
> articles on the Web and soy and phyto-estrogens are controversial, so I checked with my doctor and then made my decision.
> I did find a ton of information at the local public library. The difference between the library and web-library—I have to wait till
> they are open; they do not always have the book you want; I
> have to be presentable in public to go there.
>
> There is a ton of info on the web—there are also many quacks
> **3** out there—just like in life, you have to decide what is real,
> whats valid and what has value FOR YOU PERSONALLY. I have
> continued in my support groups on line and now help other
> newly diagnosed women. The internet is one of the greatest
> resources of our times. (E-mail 2)

Later in the book I introduce a definition of a story, and show how the above kind of account has the key characteristics of a "story" or a "narrative." It starts with an exposition of what provoked the events described (section marked as 1). Next is a description of the constellation of events, embedded in time and space, constituted by causal configuration of the different events into a whole (section marked 2). Finally there is a conclusion (section marked 3). All the sections follow the definitions of a narrative provided by Somers (1994) and Polkinghorne (1991) as further discussed in Chapter 2.

Receiving participants' e-mail replies in the form of a story was a major factor in the decision to focus on storytelling as a significant process in patients' online communication. Clearly, it was in accordance with the prominence of this discursive form on breast cancer-related online forums such as message boards and personal home pages. However, the breast cancer online environment is characterized by diverse communicative forms and processes, of which narrative and storytelling are only one. In the context of this study and its research experience, storytelling appeared as the most central of patients' communicative processes, and thus worthy of exploration.

I chose twenty-nine accounts that were rich enough in terms of both length and content for the purposes of analysis (see Appendix 1). These e-mail accounts constitute the preliminary data of the research, as they provided initial access to participants' constructions of their experience of online participation in relation to their illness.

The data collected at this stage, which is the basis for the empirical research that follows, suffers from a self-selection bias, for instance, the absence of negative accounts such as those of patients who failed to use the Internet for illness-related purposes. However, this kind of bias should be understood as a token of a broader picture of the online colloquy on breast cancer and, more generally, of the public discourse of breast cancer, the latter being about "living with breast cancer rather than dying from it" (Sharf, 1997, p. 73). As Sharf (p. 78) rightly concludes: "breast cancer talk on the Internet is a self-directed rhetoric of hope and enablement."

Moving From Online to Offline

So, the empirical process started in the online space. Obtaining participants' constructions of their experience of online participation was carried out completely by and through the Internet. However, the need for more ethnographic context implied that the research should be extended into the offline context and that accounts of participants' online experience should be obtained also offline. More specifically, given the theoretical focus on participants' storytelling online as a key process through which participants constitute themselves as agents (as discussed in the following chapter), it appeared necessary to gain some insight into their offline contexts. How do the online experience of storytelling, and the stories patients produce (or seek to produce) online, connect (or not) to their offline realities?

However, obtaining ethnographic data from patients' daily lives is highly problematic from a reflexive, feminist ethical standpoint, to which the current study subscribes. The reality of these patients is not simply "out there," at my (the researcher's) disposal, for interpretation. Hypothetically, to examine whether and how the stories patients tell online connect to their lives would involve following them in their everyday contexts, in sites such as their homes, with friends, their medical encounters and their face-to-face support groups. Observing participants in this manner appeared highly inappropriate, insensitive and impractical in the context of this study, which involves an experience that is extremely intimate and sensitive.

To maintain a reflexive ethical stance, it seemed most appropriate to rely on the accounts patients produced (in the research situation, through e-mail and face-to-face interviews, and with each other in online interaction) as data. The main offscreen method employed in this study was qualitative interviewing.[4] This was geared towards mapping and understanding the respondents' life-world frameworks, and more specifically the relation between their action (online participation) and their situation (chronic illness).

Face-to-Face Interviews

The individualistic character of patients' Internet use and online participation, along with the private nature of the illness experience, led to the decision to conduct individual interviews, rather than, for example, focus groups. I conducted twelve face-to-face, open in-depth interviews lasting between one and a half and two hours. The interviews were designed to create a situation where patients are invited to construct and recount their story. In this sense, storytelling was employed as a methodological strategy. That is, beyond a methodological means to elicit data (patients' accounts), the interview situation itself constituted part of the data; it provided a site where patients engage in storytelling.

Because the interview is treated as a storytelling site, the research experience often becomes part of the data that is being analyzed; so the empirical process itself, and the particular relationship that emerged between me (the listener) and my informants (the storytellers), enlightened in significant ways the actual phenomenon being studied. The recruitment of the face-to-face interviewees was based on the initial contacts with online participants, that is, women with whom I had been corresponding via e-mail. I contacted fifteen of the women who had replied to my message, with most of whom I had maintained correspondence since their first response, asking if they would agree to meet me for a face-to-face interview to follow up their written story in greater depth. Elsewhere I discuss at length the consideration and implications of the move from online to offline relationships with informants (Orgad, 2005a).

Analysis of the Data

The twelve face-to-face interviews constitute the core data in the analysis. In addition, I analyzed the e-mail accounts and the one received by snail mail, as well as online texts from breast cancer websites. All sources cited from the World Wide Web were last accessed in June 2004. A complementary text I analyzed is a fictional account, entitled *Dear Stranger, Dearest Friend* (Katz Becker, 2000), of an e-mail correspondence between two breast cancer patients who "met" on an online message board. Given that this is a fictional text, and thus has a different value from that of the other texts obtained through ethnography, I treated it as secondary data. Although fictional, it was nevertheless useful in illuminating the nature of e-mail correspondence that breast cancer patients may be engaged in.

In my analysis I attempted to combine the different texts rather than treating e-mail, face-to-face accounts, and website texts separately. Also, no hierarchy is implied among the different texts; all three kinds of text are treated equally in terms of their contribution to the data analysis. I used the discourse analysis of website texts to contextualize patients' e-mail and face-to-face accounts of their online experience, and vice versa. The discourse analysis of website texts is rooted in the everyday meanings that participants have of their interactions, as they emerged from their face-to-face and e-mail accounts. For example, a common feature was that, in their interviews, participants understated or even denied posting their personal stories online, but their e-mail accounts and the websites they visited showed that, in fact, they had done so.

A Note on Ethics

The ethical issues involved in conducting online studies are among the most contested areas in Internet research (Elgesem, 2002; Jankowski and van Selm, 2001; Johns, Chen and Hall, 2004). Clearly, the field is currently in a formative phase and firm guidelines for Internet researchers have yet to emerge.[5] As far as possible, I followed existing guidelines and learnt from what has been done to date. However, there were many gray areas. Ultimately, my ethical decisions were based on my personal judgment within the specific context concerned. Likewise, those decisions should be judged within the context in which they were made.

I treated participants' personal accounts with the strictest anonymity and confidentiality. During the analysis of the data, all possible appropriate precautions were taken to protect the participants' confidentiality. In quoting from face-to-face interviews I assign a number to the interview and refer to the interviewee by a letter. When quoting from e-mail interviews, only the e-mail number is indicated, avoiding any reference to the author's real e-mail address. Although the online colloquy on breast cancer forums does not constitute the main data for this research, some reference to those discussions is included in the analysis. This was done in such a way as to avoid there being any identifying links between the quotations and their respective sources. I made efforts to contact individuals who had posted messages that I wished to quote from, in order to seek their consent. However, if consent could not be obtained, I still used material from postings I considered significant and salient to be worth the risk. In such cases, I attempted to provide as much as possible the context in which the text was communicated. To disguise the original source, I edited text such that it exemplified what it was meant to, while being virtually untraceable.

When I quote from personal texts posted on online forums (personal home pages, message boards, etc.), I deliberately leave out URLs. Furthermore, in treating these online postings, the perspective I take is sociological rather than psychological. I am not interested in an individual's specific story, only in what it represents and in how it enlightens our understanding of the social and cultural context of the phenomenon under scrutiny.

At the outset, the participants in the research were informed of its aims and purposes and told that they might be quoted. I have made every effort to affect the participants, and especially those whose online and offline stories I have incorporated into this book, as little as possible.

Theoretical Context

This book suggests a new model for understanding online communication, namely storytelling online, but it is not written in a theoretical vacuum. The account I present of participants' engagement online as storytelling responds to several aspects of the existing research agenda, in particular the debate on health online and the absence of discussion on storytelling in studies of the Internet and CMC. The following section provides a brief critique of the core research agenda that includes these issues. It provides the background for the exploration of storytelling in patients' online communication.

Health Online

The proliferation of Internet use by breast cancer patients in relation to their illness is part of the broader phenomenon of the increasing use of the Internet for health-related purposes. For instance, seventy-three million adult Americans (i.e., 62% of Internet users in the United States) have turned to Internet sources of health information (Pew Internet & American Life, 2002a). According to a recent study, 24% of the Internet users who dealt with a major illness said that using the Internet was crucial to coping with it (Pew Internet & American Life, 2002b).[6]

A few years ago Burrows, Nettleton, Pleace, Loader and Muncer (2000) decried the scarcity of empirical studies about health and the Internet. Today, health-related research on CMC seems to flourish across disciplinary boundaries. More and more researchers seem to be acknowledging the potential role of the Internet in the context of health (e.g., Ferguson, 1996; Rice and Katz, 2001; Whitten, 2001). They explore the role the Internet plays in communication among health professionals (physician–physician interaction) and patients (patient–

patient communication), as well as its impact on the interaction between professionals and patients (e.g., Hardey, 1999; Reents, 1999). A review of the research agenda is beyond the scope of this book, but is provided at length elsewhere (e.g., Rice, in Rice and Katz, 2001). Within this agenda, this study relates to the work on patients' online communication.

Patients' online communication. One of the major reasons motivating patients to go online and participate is information seeking. By allowing patients access to an increasing range of information about their illness and its treatment, the Internet becomes a key actor in the transformation of the medical landscape (Bury, 2001, p. 268). Closely related to the broader agenda of the sociology and psychology of health and illness, "e-patients" (a term I am unsympathetic with, for reasons I will discuss later) are depicted as active, informed health consumers. The notion of empowerment overrules the debate: drawing on the equation "information (or knowledge) is power," studies reproduce similar findings about how the use of the Internet empowers patients (e.g., Ginossar, 2002; Millard and Fintak, 2002; Pew Internet & American Life, 2002a, 2003); how patients challenge physicians with the information they obtain online; how patients "shop around" to ensure they get the best medical service and so on.

Another much discussed aspect of the use of the Internet for patient communication is online support groups (Rice, in Rice and Katz, 2001). This aspect has been explored in numerous studies of different online contexts in which patients engage (e.g., *Alzheimer*, King and Moreggi, 1998; *Knee injuries*, Preece and Ghozati, 2001; *HIV*, Reeves, 2000; *Breast cancer*, Sharf, 1997; Shaw, McTavish, Hawkins, Gustafson and Pingree, 2000). In addition to the information-seeking aspect, those studies highlight the significance of the emotional support and affirmation that patients can receive from participating in online support groups.

Given the prominence of the Internet in relation to health, there is a case for building up a body of research on the various contexts and ways in which patients make use of the Internet. As the data analysis in this study shows, both information seeking and emotional/social support are central to patients' online experience. However, the limitation of most of the existing studies of these aspects is that they replicate findings across various patient-related online contexts. The claims they make are usually general, hackneyed and obvious: that "patients use the Internet to share information, express their feelings and offer support." The majority of the studies on patients' online communication that I found emerge from abstract typologies of patients' activities. Often written from a psychological perspective, but in some cases also using sociological thinking, they are divorced from a broader cultural and social contextualization such as the cultural meanings of the specific health context they examine. Patients' online experiences are often depicted as independent of the social and cultural relations and practices in which they are embedded. As a result, these accounts present overly functional categories to explain patients' experiences, for example, "emotional support," "esteem support," "informational support" (Shaw et al., 2000), "exchange of information," "social support" and "personal empowerment" (Sharf, 1997). While these categories seek to characterize patients' communications, too often they remain abstract generalizations that do not say what patients actually do online and what their activities mean for their lives. Unsurprisingly, in describing patients' experience, this kind of research often employs terms such as "e-patients" (Pew Internet & American Life, 2003) or "e-health" (Hardey, 2001; Whitten, 2001), as if patients' experiences existed only in relation to their online participation. In short, what is beyond the realm of "e-health" is left unexplored.

This limitation arises partly because the methodologies used to explore patient communication are often quantitative and rather mechanistic (e.g., Boyer, Provost and Baujard, 2002; Pew Internet & American Life, 2002a, 2002b, 2003). They fail to inquire into patients' perceptions of their Internet use and online experiences and the meanings of those aspects for patients' lives. In other cases, where a more integrated approach is suggested and researchers do take account of patients' perceptions (e.g., Shaw et al., 2000), they often tend to take patients' views at face value. Consequently, the analysis they produce is mostly a thematic organization of what patients said about their experience of Internet use. For instance, when discussing breast cancer patients' online communication, Shaw et al. (2000, p. 142) explain that the primary benefit of asynchronous communication is that women with conflicting schedules do not have to coordinate their schedules to chat at a specific time. This finding unquestionably derives from users' actual experience (based on interviews the researchers conducted); however, the authors remain at this purely functional level of explanation. They do not attempt to elicit a more critical account of the social processes in which those patients engage, and the potential significance of the asynchronous nature of their communication for those processes. In Chapters 5, 6 and 7, I discuss at length how the aspect of asynchronous communication is embedded in patients' experience and how it is constituted in the relationship between their offline and their online experiences.

The effect of the limitations discussed above is that a substantial part of existing literature on patients' use of the Internet is isolated from the wider critical debate on CMC. Much of the research is done within rigid disciplinary boundaries and fails to assimilate a wider critical thinking about CMC. This kind of research is often conducted for and funded by specific health organizations, which tends to direct the inquiry towards measuring aspects such as the effectiveness of the communication, or the reliability and accuracy of the information provided. As a consequence, such research tends to inquire in a very limited way (if at all) into the communicative and social dimension of patients' online experience. Indicatively, features such as anonymity, lack of social context cues and disembodiment are treated as variables in correlation with other variables such as "social support," "psychological support" and "decision making." The following statement is typical of this positivistic approach: "characteristics of the medium allowed users to manage their interactions with respect to expressiveness, stigma and obligations" (Rice, in Rice and Katz, 2001, p. 25, referring to a study by Walther and Boyd, 2002).

A more critical engagement with the data is missing from much of the literature. For research to be significant and relevant it must account for features such as "anonymity" or "disembodiment" as communicative potentials of the online space, rather than as technical properties. Categories such as "social support" should not stand as independent of features such as "anonymity." They should be integrated into an understanding of patients' communication as a process, in which they draw (or not) on certain features of the medium to accomplish their social projects. The questions that follow from such an approach are: (1) how patients' online participation connects (or not) to their offline experiences; and (2) what the relationship is between patients' online social processes and broader offline cultural and social processes (based on Slater, 2002).

The online communication of breast cancer patients. Relatively few studies have been conducted specifically on breast cancer patients' use of the Internet (Fogel, 2002, 2004; Lieberman and Russo, 2002; Pitts, 2004; Shaw, 2000; Shaw et al., 2000) and they generally suffer from the limitations that characterize the literature on patients' online communication in general. The pioneer study on breast cancer patients' online communication, and probably the most useful one, is Sharf's (1997) study of the Breast Cancer List, an online mailing list for breast cancer patients and their caregivers. This is a highly descriptive study; however, given that it was among the first written in this context, it provides a good basis for examining breast cancer online communication in a more critical fashion. Sharf (1997) takes a functional and rather simplistic approach to patients' participation in the Breast Cancer List. Based on her participant-observation in this forum she identifies three main functions of the list for its participants: exchange of information, psychological support and personal empowerment. Very little is said about the specificity of the online context for patients' experience. When Sharf addresses this aspect, she does so by comparing the online forum to face-to-face support groups. In so doing, Sharf is deterministic as she assumes a necessary difference, if not separation and opposition, between patients' online and offline experiences. She deduces, from the different properties of online and offline communication, that patients' actual experience would be substantially different. Lieberman and Russo's (2002) study has the same pitfall. In considering breast cancer online groups as a variant of face-to-face support groups, the authors attempt to isolate specific conditions of the online "group culture."

Shaw et al.'s (2000) study, which is perhaps the most significant study of breast cancer patients' CMC to date, is yet another piece of research that exhibits those inadequacies. Although it focuses on patients' experiences allegedly from "an existential phenomenological approach," it actually ignores how participants experience the Internet and the social meanings that are embedded in their experience. One of the key reasons for this is the actual design of their study. The study examines a system ("CHESS") that is installed in people's houses after they have received formal training about how to use it, and which is monitored by a facilitator. This creates a completely different setting from that of patients who use the Internet. The CHESS system appears like a deus ex machina introduced into patients' lives, as does the experience of using it. The analysis depicts an experience that is separated from, rather than integrated with, patients' everyday lives. Significantly, neither this last study, nor those mentioned above, take into account the wider cultural and social context of breast cancer such as public discourses of breast cancer in which patients' online experience is arguably embedded.

In focusing on storytelling in patients' online experience, this book attempts to draw on these existing studies while simultaneously addressing the criticisms made above. That is, it seeks to treat patients' online communication as a complex social process that is embedded in significant ways in certain social and cultural relations; to enquire into patients' views of their experience and analyze them in a critical fashion; to highlight what patients actually do online and to try to throw light on the question of why does it matter. Storytelling, I argue, seems a viable and helpful approach to examine participants' online activity, and to possibly overcome some of the shortcomings of the "e-health" debate.

Storytelling and patients' CMC. The issue of storytelling is given little attention in research on patients' CMC, and few scholars have studied it so far (Eley, 2003; Hardey, 2002; McLellan, 1997; Orgad, 2004). Hardey (2002) is perhaps the most prominent of the researchers who address the issue of narrative storytelling in the context of patients' online communication. Focusing on personal home pages of ill people, Hardey demonstrates how those online spaces constitute sites for patients' ongoing relation of their experience of illness. He draws on key ideas in medical sociology about illness narratives to illuminate a significant aspect of patients' online communication that is often and easily neglected.

However, Hardey's account is problematic in the same way as the accounts mentioned earlier. It regards the "offline" experience as the baseline for the investigation of its online "version." For Hardey, patients' online narratives are simply a novel form of traditional written illness narratives. Along the lines of structuralist analyses of traditional illness narratives, he suggests his own typology of online illness narratives. Such a typology, however, appears unhelpful in improving understanding of people's experience of Internet use in the context of their illness. McLellan (1997), too, in her study of the electronic narrative of a child diagnosed with leukemia, is concerned with establishing the differences between "conventional" health and illness narratives and online illness narratives. My experience of attending to breast cancer patients' voices has shown that patients' experiences of storytelling online should not necessarily be explained in relation to traditional forms of narrative construction. Rather, I would like to suggest, patients' online communication, particularly storytelling, in the context of this study, can be seen to be embedded in a wider culture of health and illness, of self-help and of storytelling.

There are also methodological problems with works such as Hardey's (2002) and McLellan's (1997). Relying merely on online interaction with their informants and drawing on their online texts has resulted in a limited understanding of the ways in which patients' engagement in storytelling online is interwoven with their everyday offline lives. More generally, restriction to online interactions with participants is a methodological strategy used widely in Internet studies (e.g., Baym, 2000; Donath, 1999). It often limits the interpretation of the context being researched (Bakardjieva and Smith, 2001; Hine, 2000).

In other studies, even if the notion of storytelling is mentioned, this is done in a very uncritical way. For example, in an e-mail message addressed to the members of the Association of Internet Researchers (Fox, 2003), Fox reported on a survey of "e-patients" conducted by Pew Internet & American Life project, saying that the most enlightening aspect of the study was "tons of wonderful/tragic/inspiring stories from all kinds of Internet users." This enlightenment, however, was not included in the official report. Participants were asked to fill in a semi-structured questionnaire, but rather than follow this format, they chose to tell stories. This aspect remains unaddressed. Instead of asking why storytelling "took over" the question-and-answer format, and what this might potentially reveal about the wider context of patients' online communication, the recent Pew report focuses on the old, familiar and far too general issues: information seeking, social support, accuracy and validity of health information online, and the popular topics of health-related online searches.

The Neglect of Storytelling in Internet Research

The neglect of storytelling as a central and interesting process in participants' online communication is not unique to the study of patients' CMC. While various models for understanding online communication as a socially meaningful activity have been developed since the 1980s, storytelling as a notion has hardly been mentioned. Where it is discussed, this is usually done in a very limited way. Denzin (1999), for instance, introduces the term "cybernarratives" as if it were an agreed and clear term that does not require any further exploration.[7] Only very recently, with the emergence of blogging as a popular subject in Internet research, has more attention been given to participants' engagement in storytelling; it will be interesting to see what research along these lines will produce.

In fact, CMC has often been depicted, whether explicitly or in more implicit ways, as a communicative context that stands in contradiction to the social activity of storytelling as we know it from our social offline lives, as highlighted by the following comment: "The internet is counternarrative, shaped in part by rumour, fantasy and mystical reverberation" (DeLillo, 2001, pp. 1–2).

Underlying this view of the Internet and CMC as "counternarrative" and "counterstorytelling" is a claim for the novelty of virtual worlds that afford the possibility of doing things differently with narrative than ordinary face-to-face language allows (Webb, 2001). Indeed, stressing its distinctive features, "cyberspace" has been often depicted as a space where narrative and storytelling cannot exist. This construction goes hand in hand with the broader view that governed much of the thinking in Internet studies, of the online space as an autonomous, self-contained "placeless place," separate from the offline social world (Miller and Slater, 2000; Slater, 2002).

This argument has been fuelled by studies that focus on the nonlinearity of "hypertexts" (e.g., Nelson, 1995, mentioned in Tabbi, 2000). The word "hypertext" has often been used with the intention of supplanting the notion of narrative as a linear, page-by-page movement from a clear beginning, through intermediate complications, to an ultimate resolution (Tabbi, 2000, p. 138). Hypertexts were depicted as challenging the presumption of linearity (with which we are familiar from our "offline" "real" world), presenting the reader with a completely different set of assumptions. Firstly, as Mitra and Cohen (1999) argue, the fundamental presumption that there needs to be a well-recognized beginning and end is problematized. In hypertexts it is impossible to determine what can be the authentic beginning of the text. Second,

> Unlike other texts...the WWW text is self-consciously intertextual, constantly inviting the reader to move to another textual node. The presumption of reading to the end is replaced by the expectation that the reader will "explore" and "surf" to follow the links that appear in the text. (Mitra and Cohen, 1999, p. 186)

As a consequence of the "overt nonlinear connections the text provides," so the argument goes, "the reader is liberated to produce whatever text the reader pleases" (Mitra and Cohen, 1999, p. 186). To put it simply, for scholars like Mitra and Cohen (1999) or Nelson (1995, paraphrased in Tabbi, 2000), there is an inherent contradiction between "cyberspace," along its particular features, and the capacity to produce a story.

Tabbi (2000) contests the celebrated nonlinearity of hypertext and the consequent conceptual separation between narrative and online space. He insists that we need to continue speaking of "narratives" (rather than hypertexts), considering them, however, in the different context of online space. For him,

> The post-print medium's difference lies not in its linearity or non-linearity as such, but in this potentially infinite connectivity in which all writing exists simultaneously with all other writing, so that one can no longer pretend to an objective position "outside" the written environment where life is increasingly lived. (p. 146)

Tabbi eschews the technologically deterministic trap of assuming an inherent contradiction between "cyberspace" and "storytelling." However, in trying to explain what is new about narrative and storytelling in this space, he seems to fall into a different trap, one that we could call the "structuralist sin." As the quote above shows, Tabbi seems to reify the online space as a monolithic space whose single significant characteristic is its multiplicity and simultaneity of sources. In light of this reductive definition, he explains narrative as an online discursive form.

While I acknowledge the novel opportunities and forms of communication that are facilitated by the distinctive features of the online space, I think that arguments like the ones mentioned above present too deterministic a view. They fail to account for participants' actual experiences of engaging in those online spaces. They attempt to specify the relationship between narrative, storytelling and online space, independently of the particular social uses in which this relationship is embedded.

This book seeks to overcome this inadequacy. Its point of departure is that the online space is a social space. To be understood, its properties must be contextualized in their social uses and relations (Slater, 2002). In the case of breast cancer patients, as will be argued throughout the book, not only is storytelling enabled and practiced by patients who engage online but it also constitutes a key process in their online communication. Recent studies of patients' online communication corroborate this observation, showing not only the possibility of storytelling in online spaces but also its centrality (Eley, 2003; Hardey, 2002). In light of this observation, the study underlines the need to pay adequate attention to the potential significance of narrating and storytelling in participants' experience.

The Story You Are About to Read

As in any story, the introduction to this book has set the scene for what follows. Chapter 2 presents storytelling as a theoretical framework for exploring participants' online communication as a meaningful and consequential activity. It starts by identifying four main ways in which participants', and particularly patients', online participation has been commonly understood. Next it presents an alternative model to account for patient-participants' online communication, namely, storytelling. I argue that although existing frameworks are relevant and interesting, they do not adequately account for breast cancer patients' online communication and its social significance. As an alternative, I introduce storytelling as a particularly useful way of illuminating the specific processes of communication in which breast cancer patients engage. In this context, the discussion also highlights storytelling as a model that enables a sensitive and critical consideration of the interface between the online and the offline.

To fully get to grips with participants' experience of storytelling online, we need to consider the wider context within which it is embedded. Chapter 3 describes the cultural and communicative context that frames and shapes, and is shaped by, patients' storytelling online. The discussion explores the culture of breast cancer in contemporary society and how it is interlinked with discourses of chronic illness and therapy. It shows how storytelling and narrative have become central in the social and cultural construction of breast cancer, and their therapeutic emphasis. These elements provide a significant backdrop for understanding breast cancer patients' storytelling online, which I explore in Chapters 4 to 6.

Chapters 4 to 6 are the analytical part of the book. In these chapters, I attempt to account for the specificity and the significance of the storytelling processes and forms that emerge in patients' online communication of breast cancer. Chapter 4 focuses on the aspect of emplotment (a term that I explain there) and the construction of closure. In it, I explore how online communication acts to give patients frameworks of meanings for the construction of their stories. The analysis examines how patients' engagement in storytelling online can be seen as a dialectical process that is coupled with the project of asserting themselves as survivors. Chapter 5 aims to highlight how the reciprocal relationships that emerge between patients online are significant for the facilitation of the production of their stories. I show how the specific ways in which patients interact with online structures of exchange enable them to engage in a process of storytelling, and how consequently this process gives them the power to cope with their new situation in life. Another key dimension that emerges from patients' online experience in general, and of storytelling in particular, is the negotiation of public and private. Chapter 6 develops this issue, demonstrating how patients' online narratives constitute a discursive site for the negotiation of the public and the private in their lives, a tension that is imbued with the dual meaning of illness as both private and public.

The inquiry in Chapters 4 to 6 is part of a broader intellectual endeavor to explore the significance of the processes, relations and communicative forms that emerge from individuals' online participation. Throughout these chapters I use storytelling as a model to understand what patients do online, and why what they do matters. However, I also acknowledge alternative ways of understanding what is going on, and discuss how framing them as storytelling is different from, and sometimes similar to, other models. In Chapter 7, the concluding chapter, I attempt to connect key issues raised in the book to the broader thinking about CMC and the Internet. The chapter uses the empirical case of patients' storytelling online to engage with the broader concern with the relationship between the Internet, communication and agency. I address the questions of how individuals' use of the Internet enables them to realize their agency and to what extent participants' engagement in storytelling online is a socially meaningful activity.

The chapter reflects on the usefulness and limitations of thinking about online communication in terms of storytelling. It discusses the consequences of employing this model for rethinking the way in which participants' online communicative activities have been understood and studied so far. Lastly, drawing on the analysis of breast cancer patients' online communication, the concluding remarks call into doubt the view of the online space as open, borderless, fluid and unstructured. I emphasize the need to acknowledge the constraints that shape participants' experiences. In particular, the discussion highlights the persistence of the cultural dimension in online communication, questioning the extent to which the nature of online communication is, as is often argued, global.

A final note on the format of this report: I use different fonts to reflect the different sources from which I quote (see Figure 1). When I quote an academic or any other published text that is not a direct part of the ethnographic material, I use the same font that I use in the report ("Goudy Old Style"), only in a smaller size. For quotes from face-to-face interviews used to build my analysis, I use an Arial font. Quotes from online texts (whether e-mail accounts from participants or texts harvested from public online forums) are in Verdana. Quotes from patients, e-mail accounts, face-to-face interviews or online postings are not corrected for grammar or spelling. The data is presented in this unedited way to respect the feelings of informants.

Figure 1 *Legend of Citations*

Font	Type of citation
Goudy Old Style font	citations from academic or other published texts of forty words or more
Arial font	citations from face-to-face interviews
Verdana font	citations harvested from public online forums

CHAPTER 2

Storytelling and Other Models of Online Communication

What do women who suffer from breast cancer do online? How can we describe the communication in which they engage? More specifically, what models or paradigms are available to explain their communicative activities? These questions are the point of departure for this chapter. It starts by identifying four main ways in which participants' online participation, particularly that of patients, has been commonly understood. It then moves on to presenting an alternative model to account for patient-participants' online communication, namely storytelling. I argue that existing frameworks, though relevant and interesting, are not sufficient to adequately account for breast cancer patients' online communication and its social significance. As an alternative, I introduce storytelling as a particularly useful way of illuminating the specific processes of communication and Internet spaces in which these participants engage.

The next part of this chapter establishes the conceptual framework of storytelling. The theoretical discussion first presents the definitions of "story" and "storytelling" with which this study works. This definition is a basis for a critical discussion of other approaches to storytelling, particularly those associated with structuralist and formalist narratology. After the discussion, another approach is introduced, stressing storytelling as a process. This leads to a key theoretical proposition that underlies the book: to shift from "story" to "storytelling." The following section explores in depth the concept of storytelling, ranging over several key conceptual strands: the hermeneutic approach to narrative, drawing primarily on Ricoeur's thesis of narrative as an interpretative process; his distinction between "lived" experience and "narrated" experience (Ricoeur, 1980, 1984); and the link between storytelling and agency. The discussion of the conceptual link between storytelling and agency leads to a consideration of the notion of interpretation as a helpful concept in accounting for patients' engagement in storytelling online.

The following section first discusses the employment of storytelling as a methodological strategy. Next, it presents the analytical framework that derives from the theoretical foundations and aims to substantiate the process of storytelling for the context of breast cancer patients' online experience. I discuss three specific dimensions, which, I suggest, constitute the process of patients' storytelling in the online context, namely: (1) emplotment and the construction of closure; (2) exchange and reciprocity; and (3) negotiation of private and public.

The chapter closes by connecting the ideas about patients' storytelling online to a critical debate on the online/offline distinction. In short, storytelling online is offered as a model for thinking about possible connections between participants' online and offline worlds, and as a critique of the separation between these two communicative realms.

Existing Frameworks for Explaining Patients' Online Communication

In what follows I discuss four models that were developed to explain the communicative activities and processes of online participants, and of patients in particular. I identify three key frameworks accounting for patients' online communication. These are (1) information seeking, (2) online communities and experience exchange and (3) self-presentation. I discuss these models in relation to patients' online communication, but it should be noted that they resonate in the broader conceptualization of CMC. I then discuss a fourth model—conversation.

The conversational model has governed the ways in which online communicative interactions (not only in relation to patients) have been understood and analyzed. As such, it has also had a significant impact on how patients' online communication has been explained up to now. I use the discussion of the online conversation model to reflect on the limitations of existing frameworks for accounting for patients' online communication. Against this backdrop, in the remainder of the chapter I present storytelling as a model that more adequately accounts for the processes of communication in which patients engage, and which might also account for processes of communication involving participants in other contexts.

Information Seeking

Information seeking is generally the paradigm most used to explain patients' online engagement. Existing studies have commonly regarded patients' motivation to go online, and consequently their actual activities, as primarily, if not exclusively, information driven (e.g., Burrows et al., 2000; Ferguson, 2002; Ginossar, 2002; Hardey, 1999). This focus derives from both qualitative research (e.g., Hardey, 2001, 2002) and quantitative surveys (e.g., Boyer, Provost and Baujard, 2002; Pew Internet & American Life, 2000, 2003) that have repeatedly corroborated the centrality and expansion of information seeking in patients' online activities. These studies aim at characterizing the population of online information seekers. They describe patterns of information seeking, and assess the impact of patients' information-seeking activities on the conduct of their lives, health and treatment, for example, on their relationships with their doctors (e.g., Reents, 1999).

Online Communities and Experience Exchange

While information seeking seems to have mainly governed the way patients' online experience has been explained, another less central model has examined the emergence of patients' online communities and the way their members engage in exchange of support, experience and emotions (e.g., Eysenbach, Powell, Englesakis, Rizo and Stern, 2004; King and Moreggi, 1998; Lieberman and Russo, 2002; Madara, 1999; Preece and Ghozati, 2001; Reeves, 2000; Sharf, 1997; Shaw et al., 2000). Following the larger body of literature on online communities, these studies explored the qualities of exchanging experience, emphasizing the networked, anonymous, disembodied and textual character of online groups. In the context of breast cancer, for example, Sharf (1997) shows how an online space such as a mailing list offers a platform for information sharing, social support and personal empowerment of patients and their caregivers.

Self-Presentation

A third framework that accounts for patients' online participation focuses on the ways in which patients engage in online spaces to present themselves and construct their self-narratives. Studies in this vein describe the online space, and particularly home pages, as a "stage on which the cycle of construction and reconstruction of the self is articulated" (Hardey, 2002, p. 43). In this framework, participants do not only seek information, they also produce knowledge about health through developing and maintaining their self-presentation in forms such as home pages (Hardey, 2002; Seale, 2001) or online journals (McLellan, 1997). While the discussion concerns individuals' self-presentation, and its performative and even exhibitionist (McLellan, 1997, p. 102) rather than "monologic" aspects, individuals' online self-presentations are seen as an attempt to connect. That is, as a way to engage in a conversation, and be part of a community with a strong intimate and affective dimension.

Conversation

The models discussed above explain patients' engagement online. However, as I mentioned at the beginning of this chapter, they are also related to a broader model that shaped the way in which online communicative interactions have been understood and analyzed till now, namely, the conversational model (Baym, 2002). While it is not distinctive to the study of patients' online communication, it does underpin much of the work done in this area. Considering these conceptual underpinnings, and the limitations of the conversational paradigm, helps us to understand the shortcomings of existing frameworks for explaining patients' online communication. This is the backdrop for this study in which I present storytelling online as a more useful way of elucidating the specific processes of patients' online communication.

The conversational paradigm was particularly influenced by the sociological Conversation Analysis (CA) tradition (Hutchby, 2001, p. 181). True, only a strand of these studies drew explicitly on the sociological model of face-to-face conversation to analyze online interactions. However, even when other types of analysis were performed, for instance discourse analysis of online interactions, the concept of conversation was an influential prism through which many researchers understood (and still do) how participants manage their online interaction.

While it is difficult to find a coherent definition in the literature of what is online conversation,[8] common to the different accounts of online conversation is that they position it (often implicitly) in relation to an idealized model of face-to-face conversation. This is a token of the broader theorization of online interpersonal relationships, especially of the early "reduced social cues" model, which is biased towards face-to-face communication (Lea and Spears, 1995). As the field of CMC research has developed, more complex approaches have been introduced. In particular, there has been a shift from concern with face-to-face as the basis for comparison in understanding CMC to a view of CMC as a cross between interpersonal and mass media (Baym, 2002). Nevertheless, the idea of face-to-face interaction as the basis for understanding online interaction, which is at the heart of the conversational paradigm, still resonates strongly in current thinking about CMC. This bias towards face-to-face communication can clearly be identified in the frameworks that were discussed earlier in relation to patients' online communication. For example, studies of online support groups and the exchanges in which patients engage have been often concerned with the question of how online support functions differently from offline support (Lieberman and Russo, 2002; Madara, 1999; Sharf, 1997). Such comparisons of face-to-face and online interactions reveal a set of features that characterize "online conversation" and distinguish it from face-to-face conversation.

First, online conversation is disembodied. Since disembodiment was often seen as an intrinsic property of the Internet, independent of the particular uses in which it is embedded (Slater, 2002), explorations often focused on essential questions about the possibility of communication without bodies or presence: What is interaction without bodies or presence? How binding is an online relationship that lacks contract or mutuality, and is based on disembodied interaction(s); and what kind of moral or political obligation can "virtual" contact compel? These kinds of questions reverberate in much of the discussion on CMC and particularly in the three frameworks describing patients' online communication that I discussed earlier. The preoccupation of the information-seeking model with questions about the trustworthiness and verifiability of online information derives from the concern with the latter's disembodied and consequently unregulated character. The incapacity to always relate the information patients find online to a specific recognized source, as in an embodied situation, raises difficult questions about the credibility of that information. Similar questions arise in the discussion on online support communities and self-presentation, where disembodiment is a determining dimension—for instance, how the lack of visual and tactile communication affects the nature of support online (Sharf, 1997, p. 74).

Second, online conversation has been commonly seen as textual rather than oral. Quite simply, it is carried on through means of typed text rather than speech (Hutchby, 2001, p. 173). The textual (disembodied) has been often equated with the impersonal and inauthentic while the oral (embodied) is depicted as the genuine and intimate. More context-sensitive models acknowledged CMC as a hybrid communicative situation, containing both oral and written characteristics (e.g., Baym, 2002; Fernback, 2003). However, they too often remain captured by the idea that the oral is the authentic, interpersonal and interactive. "Like speech," explains Baym (2002, p. 65), "much CMC is direct, contextualized and interactive," implying that the textual is necessarily not all these things. So even when accounting for CMC as entailing oral qualities, the sense has been usually of restoring an idealized face-to-face interaction. In the context of "e-health" research, for example, in the self-presentation paradigm, both McLellan's (1997) and Hardey's (2001, 2002) studies of patients' online narratives focus on the textual properties of these self-disclosures. Their concern is mainly with the texts that patients produce online, rather than the processes in which these texts come into being. While these processes are followed through the typed text rather than speech, I argue that at the same time they display significant oral qualities of talking and chatting. The social significance of "e-health" interactions cannot be fully understood when the hybrid character of online communication as both textual and oral is not recognized.

Another corollary of the comparison between CMC and an idealized model of face-to-face conversation is the stress on the lack of control of participants in online conversation. In face-to-face conversation the exchange has been often portrayed as one that "can be straightforwardly managed" by the participants (Hutchby, 2001, p. 186), and allows them a high degree of control. Online exchanges are understood as the reverse. Consequently, accounts exploring online conversation have focused on the challenges that participants face in online conversation. What kinds of controls and intermediaries that do not exist in a face-to-face context are present online, and how do participants deal with them? What are the implications of the incapacity of participants to choose and to fully control the different elements of the communicative interaction (their partners, the time, place and topic of the conversation)? The notion of control, or rather participants' lack of it, has been very pertinent in the discussion on information seeking online. For example, the question of whether health seekers trust the online prescription marketplace (Pew Internet & American Life, 2004) is, in broader terms, a question about the degree of control participants exercise online compared to what they enjoy in the offline institutionalized prescription marketplace. Accounts of online support groups and patients' self-presentation often address the question of control by comparing the capacity of online participants to manage their interactions with fellow sufferers, caregivers and health professionals with their capacity to do so in offline interactions (e.g., Lieberman and Russo, 2002; McLellan, 1997; Sharf, 1997).

Online conversation has also often been depicted as lacking coherence. Drawing closely on the CA perspective, textual online conversation has been claimed to be interactionally incoherent due particularly to two obstacles in the properties of the medium: low degree of adjacency (messages are posted in the order received by the system without regard for what they are responding to) and reduced feedback (lack of audiovisual cues and the fact that messages cannot overlap; Herring, 1999). While these characteristics were based mainly on studies of synchronous environments, the claim about the incoherence of online conversation applies to online interaction more generally and also in asynchronous settings. Thus, patients' online narratives are described by Hardey (2002) and McLellan (1997), for example, as unruly, hybrid and unfinished, in comparison to their written offline counterparts, which are supposedly more coherent and have a closure.

The model of online conversation throws light on how participants manage their interactions at the interface between the norms of conversation and the communicative properties of the online space. In the context of this study, the conversational model and the three other models that account for patients' online communication have much to offer for understanding breast cancer patients' online communication. As stated earlier and as later chapters will show, one of the central aspects of patients' online engagement is the search for health information. Another meaningful activity is exchange of personal experience with fellow sufferers. The model of self-presentation can shed light on the ways in which breast cancer patients engage in the online construction of their identities.

That being said, these models suffer from several limitations, and so are limited in their capacity to explain the context of the study described in this book. The first drawback to the conversational paradigm is that it does not allow enough room for communicative processes and practices that are not necessarily dialogic or interactive. In the context of their online communication, I suggest that there is a range of activities and processes in which breast cancer patients engage that cannot be explained by the notions of "conversation," at least not as they are defined by the conversational paradigm. While the reciprocal dimension plays a central role in patients' online communication, as I explore in Chapter 5, there are also significant noninteractive processes that need to be accounted for, such as lurking, for example. However, the conversation model overlooks such processes.

A second inadequacy of the conversational model (and by extension of the other models to a large degree) is that it conceives online conversation as a constrained version of face-to-face embodied conversation, which is implicitly elevated to the supreme status of idealized communicative interaction. While traditional Conversation Analysis depicts face-to-face conversation as a dialogic, embodied, private, authentic and controlled interaction, it is cast in opposition to the disembodied, public, inauthentic online conversation. As a consequence, whether celebrating the capacity of participants to empower themselves by connecting with others and experiencing their identity in new ways—online communication as re-authenticity—or decrying the loss of "real," "genuine" communication, as in the infamous case of the cross-dressing psychiatric (Stone, 1995)—online communication as de-authenticity, the underlying agenda has been the need to restore a dialogic relationship of body to body, the latter likened to authenticity.

Recent research casts a critical light on the concern with authenticity, suggesting that the question should not be whether online interaction is more or less authentic than "real" interaction, but rather where, when and how these interactions are made available on the Internet (Hine, 2000, p. 118). The account of patients' storytelling online in this book sheds critical light on how existing models equate (however implicitly) face-to-face embodied and oral interaction with authenticity, depicting online disembodied textual interactions as necessarily less authentic or less "genuine." I claim that patients' storytelling online, conducted in a disembodied, textual fashion, is highly meaningful for its participants. In the context of my study, I suggest that rather than asking whether patients' online interactions are "authentic," it seems more appropriate to focus on the question of how online interactions are experienced as social processes that are meaningful for the participants.

Finally, the fascination with the novel and distinctive characteristics of online conversation, of disembodiment, textuality, virtuality and anonymity, has often led to a tendency to regard the online space as being apart from social life and disconnected from the offline realm (Slater, 2002). Although many studies go to great lengths to characterize the experiences and processes of information seeking online, they rarely consider the everyday experiences of the seekers, or account for the wider social and cultural context of health and illness that surrounds online information seeking. Much of the research on patients' experiences of online exchanges and support groups fails in the same way. How the phenomenon can be explained in light of the wider culture of self-help and self-therapy and how the sharing of emotions online affects participants' capacity to cope with their illness are the kinds of questions that often remain unexplored. Consequently, claims about the social significance of information seeking, online community, exchange and self-presentation appear limited and unsustainable. A key endeavor of this book in developing storytelling as a model to account for patients' online communication is to demonstrate how this communicative context is interlinked with, rather than separated from, the offline domain. I elaborate this point later in this chapter.

This book offers a different model for understanding what participants do online, namely storytelling. This does not mean that I dismiss the usefulness of other frameworks. Rather, I argue that storytelling is a particularly useful way of illuminating the specific processes of communication and Internet spaces in which breast cancer patients engage. As the book progresses, it will become evident that in some aspects the proposed model of storytelling intersects with other models. For instance, in Chapter 5 I explore the centrality of exchange processes and the communal aspect in patients' storytelling online. Yet in other senses, storytelling is developed as a way of challenging and critiquing existing ways of looking at online communication.

In short, in presenting storytelling as a framework for understanding participants' online communication as a socially meaningful activity, I highlight both the strengths and the weaknesses of alternative existing models. The concluding chapter reflects on the benefits and the limitations of employing storytelling as a model for our broader thinking on online communication. I now introduce the conceptual framework of storytelling online, which I employ in the exploration of patients' online communication in Chapters 4 to 6.

Storytelling: An Introduction

Breast cancer patients seem often to express themselves on online spaces such as message boards or journals in narrated forms, which they refer to as "stories":

> I wish someone would listen to my *story* (A title of a message posted on a breast cancer message board [italics added])

> If there was no Internet, I might have chosen to tell the *story* of cancer and coping through lectures and talks with other patients. (E-mail 3 [italics added])

> I shared my *stories* on several sites and wondered which site that you read my *story* on? (E-mail 13 [italics added])

When we say that patients exchange stories in online spaces, at first sight, the notions of "story" and "storytelling" seem obvious. We are familiar with the concept of storytelling on an intuitive basis, from the experience of our everyday life. Indeed, the centrality of storytelling to individuals' everyday lives is a theoretical supposition underlying this book.

However, beyond its commonsensical meaning, the concept of storytelling carries multifaceted and complex intellectual baggage. Given the ample scope of the concept and its extensive and enduring study, a pertinent preliminary task is to define what is meant by storytelling in this study, specifically in relation to breast cancer patients' online experience.

A useful entry point to this task is an actual example of a text that was posted by a breast cancer patient on an online message board:

> When I was diagnosed last November, it was already too late. I found a lump in my left breast last summer. I had benign lumps in my breast for years. Normally they went away after some days. So I thought this time, and forgot them. In September I noticed the lump again. It even was a bit bigger. I went to my doctor who told me not to care. In october the lump was nearly twice as big as the lump I first found in July. My doctor still said I do not have to care, the lump is benign and will disappear from alone. In November I moved to a different town, so I had no time to think about the lump. Late in December, I found the lump was much bigger now. But as Christmas was coming, there was no time, too, and I wanted no illness. Things got worse in January. I awake one morning with my breast red and swollen. I was shocked when I saw little ulceration down the breast. My new doctor was shocked when he saw me. He told me after some test that I have terminal inflammatory breast

> cancer and only a few months left. It was a shock for me, too, finding out that there is a large cancer killing me. It had already spread to my lung, liver, intestines and bladder.... I get palliative care. Morphium for pain.... Is getting worse. The tumor is growing very fast. My doctor never saw such a fast growing. The skin ulceration of my breast is getting larger. Half of the skin is ulcerated, and the tumor inside my breast nearly fills it. I am getting skin metastasis in my axilliary and around my belly button.... I am angry that I did not see a doctor last Summer and forced him to look closer.

This online text is clearly a story. The author reorganizes the course of her illness as a chain of events, ordered clearly along a timeline. The temporal ordering allows the author to make sense of her experience: to organize people, events and information that she encountered, into a coherent framework of meaning. Events that were "objectively" disconnected from the experience, such as Christmas or moving to a different town, are incorporated into a coherent story. The above text could therefore be described as a narrative or a story:[9] "[A] constellation[s] of *relationships* (connected parts) embedded in *time* and *space*, constituted by *causal emplotment*" (Somers, 1994, p. 616, italics in original).

Implied in this definition of narrative, as is evident in the text cited above, is that we can "discern the meaning of any single event only in temporal and spatial relationship to other events" (Somers, 1994, p. 616). In other words, narrative renders understanding only by connecting parts to a constructed configuration. When the author writes, "I awake one morning" the meaning of "one morning" can be fully grasped only in relation to the events that preceded it.

Storytelling is the attempt to produce a framework to organize disconnected elements into a whole and direct them toward closure. In narrative study this process is often referred to as emplotment: the procedure that configures the different events into a whole by grasping them together and directing them toward a conclusion or ending, thereby giving significance to independent instances (Polkinghorne, 1991; Somers, 1994, based on Ricoeur, 1984). Through emplotment, the author is able to construct a significant configuration of relationships between the different instances: she organizes her story along all the alarming moments she had ignored, relating each to a specific month in the year. Her online story constitutes a framework that configures different events, actions and experiences into a plot, through which she tries to make sense of her illness. Hardey (2002) describes a similar process in his examination of patients' personal home pages, for instance, in the online story of Teresa, a patient diagnosed with Hodgkin's disease: "Like the other accounts provided on the home pages Teresa's narrative is given a coherence and order by the way that events are linked together retrospectively within a broadly sequential framework" (p. 36).

From Story to Storytelling, From Text to Process

In employing this definition of storytelling to explore patients' online communication, and particularly in emphasizing the process rather than the text, this study seeks to move beyond structuralist perspectives of narratives (most associated with the work of Lévi-Strauss, 1968, and Barthes, 1977) and the formalist narratology, which is primarily indebted to Vladimir Propp (1968). Structural approaches stress the form as taking precedence over the content (Lévi-Strauss, 1968, p. 204). In so doing, they underscore the universal, ubiquitous and eternal nature of stories. At the same time, however, they fail to explain their ubiquity, that is, to reveal their significance (Gare, 2002, p. 93). Their exclusive concern with narrative as a form overlooks the process in which narrative is being configured and the meaning of this process for individuals' everyday social lives.

Media studies have predominantly followed the structuralist and formalist path in their exploration of the relation between media and stories. The chief focus has been on exploring the narrative qualities of different media texts, for example, news (Bird and Dardenne, 1988), television documentary programs (Silverstone, 1983, 1984, 1988)[10] and advertising (Berger, 1997; Kozloff, 1992). They used the analysis of media as narrative to shed light on the wider values, symbols and meanings that exist in contemporary culture. As Kozloff (1992, p. 69) expressed it: "Narratives are not only the dominant type of text on television, but narrative structure is, to a large extent, the portal or grid through which even nonnarrative television must pass."

Despite the significance of structuralist analyses of media narratives, a question that remains unanswered is why those stories, being told by and through the media, matter: how those stories have come into being; where they come from in terms of their history, organization and the influence of specific individuals; and what psychological and social consequences they have both for their audience and for their producers (Kozloff, 1992). Kozloff (1992), who uses a Proppian analytical framework for her study, herself admits to some limitations in this approach. The shortcomings of the structuralist approach to narrative and its merits can be seen in studies of online illness narratives. Along a similar line to the brief analysis of a patient's online text presented above, McLellan (1997) and Walstrom (1999) demonstrate in great detail how texts that patients post online contain the structural elements of narrative. They highlight how narrative elements such as the author's positioning as a protagonist (see Walstrom, 1999) are employed by participants in their online representation. However, this line of analysis is limited in its capacity to reveal the specificity and significance of those mediated stories and their consequences for both their tellers and listeners. For one, as Hardey (2002) notes, many of the narrative elements that appear in patients' online texts have been described in earlier research on illness narratives.

Therefore, for the purpose of examining breast cancer patients' processes of online communication, this book seeks to move beyond a structuralist perspective and an analysis of stories as structures. It suggests that, in examining breast cancer patients' online communication, it is useful to shift the focus from stories to storytelling. That is to say, the subject of this study is not patients' online texts as narrative forms, but rather patients' work of making those texts online and its significance for their lives. In this formulation, the emphasis is not on the final product but on the struggle to produce it, that is, to produce a framework that will organize disconnected elements into a whole and direct them toward closure.

So storytelling is more than simply self-disclosure or sense making and less than a fixed, delimited text. It lies in the middle ground between the two. Hence the exploration of storytelling falls neither in the domain of literary analysis, which is concerned with the textual properties of narrative, nor in the psychiatric domain, whose focus is the process of confession. Storytelling is about an attempt to communicate one's experience to others, including strangers, by ordering it in time and gearing it to a closure. This process might materialize into the production of a story—a delimited textual form that orders experience in time and directs it toward closure. It might, at the same time, not involve the actual creation of a final product (story) but still occupy a meaningful process, in that it allows participants to attempt to make sense of their experience in a certain way.

At the heart of the inquiry into patients' storytelling online are questions about the significance of the production and telling of a story in patients' online experience; how this process affects patients' ways of being and how the stories patients seek to produce and tell online enable them to act. The next section constitutes the theoretical foundation for addressing the above questions. It aims to clarify and qualify the theoretical assertions that will later inform the analysis of the data on breast cancer patients' online communication.

Storytelling: Theoretical Foundations

The theoretical framework of this book is predicated upon the tradition of hermeneutics that views storytelling as a continuing interpretation and reinterpretation of experience, rather than as a record of what happened. In particular, Ricoeur's seminal thesis of the relationship between time and narrative is of key importance.

For Ricoeur (1980, 1984) narrative is the fundamental structure of the experience of time. It is the only temporal form that succeeds in capturing the sense of lived time. Unlike clock or calendar time forms, for example, narrative bears a mimetic relationship to experience as lived. The mimesis in narrative is threefold, that is, it consists of three moments: prefiguration, configuration and refiguration (Gare, 2002, p. 94). First, there is a preunderstanding of the world as action. At this stage there is a symbolic system that furnishes a descriptive context for particular actions (Ricoeur, 1984, p. 58). The second moment of mimesis involves the representation of action according to specific rules of emplotment: the making of a structure that configures the preunderstanding. This "configurational arrangement transforms the succession of events into one meaningful whole" and "imposes the 'sense of ending' on the indefinite succession of incidents" (p. 67). This moment of emplotment "opens the kingdom of the *as if*" (p. 64, italics in original). The third moment is the appropriation and actualization of the structure (the plot). It is the moment where the world of the text (the structure) and the world of the hearer or the reader (action) intersect (p. 71). In short, through the configuration of experience into a narrative, "people are provided with room to maneuver, to think about how they construe the way they live, which allows them to refigure their lives by appropriating new structures" (Gare, 2002, p. 94). Implicit in this observation is a fundamental recognition of the inextricable relation between storytelling and agency. The next section unfolds the concept of agency and discusses its relation to storytelling.

The concept of agency and its link to storytelling. The ability to make sense of experience and construct a plausible story that can be incorporated into one's life is a requisite for one's agency, that is, one's capacity to act. Agency emerges from the capacity of individuals, in this case, breast cancer patients, to project and think utopically, beyond the constraints of their conditions, and so to "elude what determines thought and imagination" (Langbauer, 1992, p. 51, cited in Gardiner, 2000, p. 17). As Lefebvre (1984, p. 75, cited in Gardiner, 2000, p. 18) asserts: "we are all utopians, as soon as we wish for something different."

The notion of agency, as construed in this study, stresses the potential for individuals to transform their existing social conditions (Gardiner, 2000). Such focus has particular significance when a disruption to the daily routine such as cancer is concerned. As actors who can no longer rely on commonsensical notions, following this disruption of what previously constituted the taken-for-granted in their lives, patients are highly receptive to alternative modes of being. It is then that the utopian moment, which is emblematic of a longing for a different and better way of living, arises.

At the same time, despite the centrality of ideas about transformative capacity, activity, creativity and potentiality in explaining patients' online engagement, in this book I try to avoid overemphasizing the resistant and utopian qualities of users' everyday practices by adopting the concept of agency. The notion of agency regards the processes in which patients are involved—in this case particularly in relation to their use of the Internet—as essentially dialectical. The view draws closely on Giddens' (1984) influential theorization of human agency. It implies that the construction of a story online is a means by which a patient can realize her transformative potential, that is, her capacity to circumvent the disturbance being imposed on her life by the cancer, and to monitor her actions. The utopian dimension is contained insofar as "Agency refers not to the intentions people have in doing things, but to their capability of doing those things in the first place" (Giddens, 1984, p. 9).

That is, patients' capacity to reflexively monitor their action should be evaluated in terms of their actual capability to act, and the constraints in which they operate. This view recognizes the significant role that different structures continuously play in the capacity to achieve desired goals. In the context of the present study, this means that it is necessary to look at the connection between patients' online activity and their offline experiences, or how participants' online engagement feeds into their capacity to act. This dialectic runs throughout this book's exploration of storytelling online as a site for the realization of patients' agency.

The link between agency and storytelling implies that, in order to realize our transformative capacity, we need to engage in the creation of stories. "It is essentially through narratives that individuals become more than the conditions of their existence" (Gare, 2002, p. 97).

Storytelling, Self-Formation and Interpretation

The hermeneutic relation between storytelling and agency suggests that, in interpreting symbolic forms, individuals incorporate them into their own understanding of themselves and others, using them as vehicles for reflection and self-reflection, as a basis for thinking about themselves and others (Thompson, 1995). Storytelling is a central process through which this self-reflection is exercised and performed. Individuals understand themselves and construct their self-identities by working and reworking their interpretations of their own biographies in the form of stories (Giddens, 1991).

So the symbolic project of the self is increasingly nourished by available mediated symbolic materials, "materials which the individual weaves into a coherent account of who he or she is, a narrative of self identity" (Thompson, 1995, p. 210). This process of interpretation and sense making (which does not necessarily have to do with the production of stories) has been widely studied by audience research in relation to the reception of media products (e.g., Ang, 1985; Hobson, 1982; Livingstone, 1998; Radway, 1987). Recently e-health studies have also addressed the issue of interpretation by patients who encountered medical information online (Eastin, 2001; Hardey, 2001; Pew Internet & American Life, 2000, 2003). In this context, however, the notion of interpretation has mainly referred to patients' understanding and evaluation of the relevance, credibility and accuracy of the health information they encounter online. This notion of interpretation is expressed in the following account of one of my interviewees:

> It takes time to know whether or not breast cancer patients have been helped or misdirected by information that they have picked up on the Internet. The most important issue, of course, is *interpretation*. (E-mail 9 [italics added])

Audience research regards interpretation as the process by which media consumers negotiate with the meanings of a media text such as a television program, while e-health studies focus on interpretation as a process by which participants critically accept and evaluate the information they encounter online.

The notion of interpretation is also very central to this research. This study centers on the process of producing a story and its telling online as a fundamentally interpretative process through which patients seek to make sense of their illness. However, the way "interpretation" is construed in this book in relation to storytelling differs from the way both audience research and e-health studies use it. It differs from the general process of interpretation and sense-making activity in audience research in that it is geared toward the production of a story. This does not mean that storytelling must result in the final product of narrative, but it definitely has to involve some kind of attempt or struggle to produce it, that is, to create a framework that would capture and integrate into a complete story multiple and scattered events, directing them toward a closure (Ricoeur, 1984). Storytelling online as an interpretative process is different from patients' interpretations in e-health studies of online information in that it is not based on a critical evaluation of the truthfulness and credibility of existing information online. Rather, it is an attempt to produce a self-story that helps its teller and her listeners to make sense of her experience. Producing such a story might involve the evaluation of the trustworthiness of other information, but this is not the purpose of this activity.

Analytical Framework: Storytelling in the Online Experience of Breast Cancer Patients

In light of the account presented so far, I suggest the online environment should be regarded as a significant space where patients try to capture the sense of "lived time" by producing and telling their personal stories, besides engaging in other activities. Breast cancer is a life-threatening disease that has fundamentally disturbed the sufferer's everyday lived experience. Consciously or not, patients are involved in a continuous attempt to control the uncontrollable, to recapture the lived experience that has been threatened by the intrusion of cancer into their lives. Under these circumstances, storytelling appears to be a way to encompass the "real time" of experience, and so capture life and gain a sense of control.

In light of the theoretical discussion provided in this chapter, the analysis of breast cancer patients' CMC focuses on patients' struggles to make sense of their experience by seeking the construction of a framework of meaning that configures their experience into a story, directing it toward some kind of ending. So the focus of the analysis is not on the final product—that is, the textual forms participants post online—but rather the processes, activities and structures that are involved in their attempt to produce a story. To further clarify: a patient might have never posted a text that qualifies as a story in the conventional sense (a delimited textual form), yet might still be engaged in a process of storytelling.

True, this kind of analysis allows the notion of storytelling to become extremely broad and ill defined, since it is not necessarily anchored to a clear fixed textual form that represents a "story" or "narrative." It implies that storytelling can embrace different utterances or discourses that contain elements of a story, yet does not constitute a narrative that can be encompassed by any conventional definition. Despite the caveats to framing patients' online experience in terms of storytelling, I suggest that this framework enlightens our understanding of the processes, practices, structures and forms involved in those patients' online experience in ways that other frameworks cannot.

Dimensions of Patients' Storytelling Online

My aim in this section is to substantiate the process of storytelling online as presented in the broad theoretical discussion, asking what kinds of things this process stands for. The dimensions represent three key aspects that characterize patients' storytelling online: emplotment and the construction of closure, exchange and reciprocity, and the negotiation of private and public. Although these are not distinctive aspects of storytelling and CMC, they emerge from the analysis as central and thus appeared helpful in framing patients' online experience.

Emplotment and the construction of closure. When a person contracts an illness such as breast cancer, how the situation will develop is largely unknown. There is no temporal horizon by which the illness can be evaluated (Hydén, 1997). While a patient's main endeavor might be regaining certainty and control, the reality of the illness does not allow final closure, as there is always the risk of recurrence.

This is the background to the discussion of emplotment and the construction of closure in Chapter 4. Certain online forms, I argue, encourage the production of patients' stories, enabling them in implicit (and sometimes explicit) ways to emplot their experience. The process of storytelling online directs the personal experiences of patients towards the construction of closure. In this sense, the online discursive domain serves to close patients' illness experience. At the same time, the dynamic unfixed nature of online communication allows users to change and revise their texts, so storytelling online also facilitates the ongoing production of an experience that has no closure.

In exploring this dimension, the discussion focuses on how storytelling online enables this dialectical process. The analysis of breast cancer patients' online communication looks at the particular elements that enable the process of constructing a story, geared towards a closure, yet allowing, as Good (1994, in Hydén, 1997) puts it, a "forever search of meaning." The analysis inquires into how specific online properties are embedded in patients' dialectical processes of survival: of closing and leaving open, of forgetting and remembering at the same time.

Exchange and reciprocity. In the online spaces of breast cancer patients, storytelling is often based on a reciprocal exchange-based interaction between tellers and listeners. The analysis of the role of exchange in patients' online experience, particularly in relation to storytelling, will be informed by several theoretical assertions that emphasize the interrelation between exchange and storytelling.

According to Brooks (1994) and Spence (1982), in order for a story to acquire a workable truth that enables the teller to cope with his/her condition, the narrative truth must be confirmed. The confirmation requires an external listener, an understanding that resonates with Bakhtin's (1984) notion of the dialogic word—for Bakhtin the word is always implicitly in a situation of exchange. The teller has to have an implicit knowledge that there is the Other who confirms the truth of her story. In psychoanalytic terms, in order for a construction of a story to succeed, it must be based on a "jointly authored work" (Schafer, 1980, p. 32). No story can ever be told in a social vacuum. Narratives "emerge in joint actions, become objects for interpretation in joint actions, and can be refashioned through joint actions" (Plummer, 1990, p. 136). This is the theoretical foundation for the analysis in Chapter 5.

Negotiating the public and the private. Another important theoretical thread that informs the analysis concerns the relations between storytelling, and the public and the private. The act of publishing a personal story in a public space such as a personal home page moves it from the private domain to the public domain.

Indeed, one of the key aspects of the illness narratives that are described in the literature is the transformation of illness from an individual into a collective phenomenon. Through narrative, the illness is removed from the private sphere and becomes a collective experience (Hydén, 1997). Through writing, the suffering of the individual can become something that is shared (Rosenblum, 2000).

Drawing on these theoretical claims, the analysis in Chapter 6 reflects on the meanings of private and public that emerge around the act of storytelling in online space.

Storytelling Online: Turning a "Full Stop" Into a "Comma"

> Do not place a period where God has placed a comma! I have tried to live my life that way. This [breast cancer] is just my comma in life. (A message posted on a breast cancer message board)

This chapter has introduced the core exploration of this book: to show how the different ways in which stories are constructed and told on the online space comprise a communicative situation that frames patients' experience of illness in profound ways. The analysis of the data along the three dimensions attempts to demonstrate how storytelling constitutes a means for patients, in their refusal to succumb to their illness, to attempt to regain the normality and mundanity of their everyday lives. The experience of the construction and the telling of a story is displayed as one way in which a patient becomes capable of turning the disruption imposed by the cancer into a mere "comma," which gives her the power to cope with her new station in life.

Figure 2 summarizes the propositions made in this chapter about the relationship between the process of storytelling online and the realization of agency:

Figure 2 *The Relationship Between Storytelling and Agency*

Storytelling ◄···························► Agency

Emplotment and construction of closure
Exchange and reciprocity
Negotiation of public and private

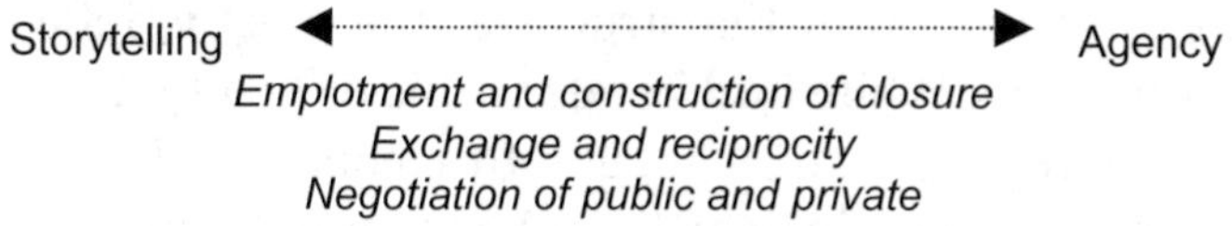

I suggest that agency and storytelling work in a dialectical relationship. The dimensions in italics are the key processes that embody this dialectical relationship. It is through the act of storytelling online that those processes are pursued and, as a consequence, a patient understands and demonstrates her capacity to act. In this sense, storytelling constitutes a main source for agency, working from the left- to the right-hand side of the diagram. At the same time, it is only when one is capable of acting, thinking beyond the constraints of one's conditions, that these projects (the italicized dimensions) can be pursued and one can engage in storytelling. Thus, storytelling is, simultaneously, the product of agency, going from the right-hand side of the diagram to its left-hand side. As Bruner (1987, pp. 12–13) puts it: "the mimesis between life so-called and narrative is a two way affair.... Narrative imitates life, life imitates narrative."

Storytelling Online at the Interface Between the Online and the Offline

The emphasis on the interlink between storytelling and agency in patients' online experience introduces the possibility of thinking about whether and how their online and offline worlds are connected. Considering patients' storytelling online as presented here assumes that a patient's offline experience, what Ricoeur terms "lived experience," provides materials that are woven into the story she produces online. In this sense, through storytelling, and particularly the second moment that Ricoeur calls "configuration," offline experiences feed into online experiences. Configuring their experience into a story online allows patients to think of themselves beyond the conditions and constraints of their lives and to appropriate the new structures they create within which to refigure their lives.

This assumption describes a clearly utopian moment. Arguably, however, it might not correspond with patients' offline lives. A patient might construct her experience into a workable framework online, but may not be capable of translating it into her everyday coping with the illness. Assuming that the moment of emplotment unproblematically leads to an actualization of the structure (the plot) is indeed a wider conceptual difficulty. While I do not deny this difficulty, I do not intend to resolve it here. My aim is to use this conceptual proposition to enlighten possible ways in which patients' storytelling online might connect to their offline worlds. In particular, how materials from their offline lives are woven into their online stories and how the stories they try to construct online help them organize a structure within which they can think and live in their offline worlds.

This line of thinking links to a wider critique of much of the existing literature on CMC and Internet use. This literature tends to posit the "online" and the "offline" as a dichotomy, regarding the online space as a space apart from social life rather than as an integral part of it. Such critique includes those raised by Baym (2000), Haythornthwaite and Wellman (2002), Hine (2000), Miller and Slater (2000), Slater (2002) and Wynn and Katz (1997), who criticized the earlier generation of Internet writing for its focus on the separation of the offline from the online, and for its assumption "that only things that happen on the Internet were relevant to understanding the Internet" (Haythornthwaite and Wellman, 2002, p. 5). The separation and dichotomization between the online and the offline are closely interlinked with the conversational paradigm that cast computer-mediated interactions in opposition to face-to-face.

Another criticism of existing studies of the Internet is that they perceive the relationship between online and offline as the relationship between phenomenon and context. Accordingly, the offline was often treated as that which makes sense, or explains, the online. As a result, "putting the online into the offline reifies both: it assumes a thing called the Internet and a thing called society, or community, or social relations, and at best investigates how one affects the other" (Slater, 2002, p. 544).

In describing patients' online experience of storytelling, this book follows this line of critique. The Internet, and thus patients' storytelling online, is seen as embedded in participants' everyday lives. My aim is to open up the possibility for thinking about storytelling as a site where the online and offline can connect. Along these lines, I purposely avoid treating the experience of breast cancer as the context for the phenomenon of storytelling online. Rather, the two are seen as contextualizing each other: women's experience of the illness provides the context for understanding their online experience, while at the same time it is a phenomenon that can be explained in light of the context of their online experience.

Underlying this integrative approach is an attempt to assess the significance of the Internet as a social phenomenon (Haythornthwaite and Wellman, 2002, p. 10). This approach has been adopted by different kinds of study. I want to briefly map two key approaches that attempt to make such connections between the online and the offline, and then locate my own study in relation to them.

One group of studies, most associated with the work of Barry Wellman (1999; Hampton and Wellman, 2003), is concerned with the effect of the Internet on individual well-being, relations with others and social capital building within communities. It explores the relationship between individuals' connection to the Internet and their online activities, and their levels of loneliness and connectivity in their local communities. The other kind of research takes an ethnographic approach to the study of the Internet. Most notable is perhaps Miller and Slater's (2000) study of the Internet in Trinidad. The authors advocate an ethnographic approach that explores the inextricable connections between "the Internet" and "society," one that sees the Internet as embedded in a specific place that it also transforms. Unlike Wellman, Miller and Slater are not interested in asking about the use and effect of the new medium. Rather, they look at how a specific culture acts and reacts in a transforming communicative environment where the Internet plays a central role.

The strength of both approaches is that they emphasize the need for serious empirical research. Claims for the inseparability of the online and the offline are being made more frequently, but they often lack anchorage in specific empirical evidence. This book similarly claims that to be able to argue for storytelling as a site where the online and the offline connect, it has to be analyzed empirically in its specificity as a social phenomenon.

Although Wellman stresses the need to consider the Internet as embedded in everyday life, the questions he asks about the impact of the Internet on the everyday start from the assumption that the two are separate. Wellman looks at the two communicative domains separately, and then establishes the connections between them, for example, the link between being wired or not, and people's informal contact with neighbors (Hampton and Wellman, 2003). Some of the surveys of the

Pew Internet & American Life Project follow similar lines, attempting to make connections between users' online and offline activities. In so doing, this kind of research to some degree maintains the dualism between the Internet and the everyday, between the online and the offline. Furthermore, the specificities and variations of Internet and online communications seem to be collapsed into a unitary "thing," namely "the Internet," whose relationships with the offline domain are then investigated.

Like Miller and Slater, but unlike Wellman and much of the e-health-type research, I am not interested here in asking about the "effect" of "the Internet" on breast cancer patients' lives. Rather, the emphasis is on the social space that is created in the intermeshing between the two communicative realms. The question that interests me is how participants engage in the communicative environment of the Internet to make sense of their lives. My starting point is that what patients do online, and storytelling in particular, is part of their everyday life. It is a process of mediation, a space where the technology—the Internet—and the social life of patients interact. So I do not examine storytelling online in comparison or in contrast to participants' "other" domains of the everyday. Unlike the work of Wellman and his research group, I do not try to establish the connections between the Internet and everyday life by collecting data on participants' online activities and patterns of use and on their offline activities and characteristics. Rather, I ask people about their experience of engaging in the online communicative space and, on the basis of their accounts as well as observation of their activity online, I try to explain the social significance of this phenomenon.

In this sense, this book is more sympathetic to the ethnographic approach advocated by Miller and Slater. However, unlike Miller and Slater, methodologically my research does not involve obtaining ethnographic material from participants' daily lives. Miller and Slater would probably argue that it is only on the basis of ethnographic evidence about patients' everyday lives outside the domain of storytelling that we can make claims about the connections and disconnections between participants' online and offline lives, and in the case of this study, between their engagement in storytelling online and their agency. Numerous studies have documented how people's construction of their fictive selves online is disconnected from their offline selves and their sense of agency (e.g., Stone, 1995; Turkle, 1996). So without exhaustive ethnographic evidence, how can I make claims about the significance of what is going on online for the way patients' manage their illness?

Despite the merit of this claim, to look for ethnographic material of patients' reality "out there," "outside" storytelling, seems inconsistent with this study's notion of storytelling. As I have discussed in this chapter, theoretically, storytelling and agency are seen as being mutually implicated, and the very act of storytelling is understood as transforming the teller. Action is assumed as being embedded within thought and discourse, rather than occurring in a separate "everyday" domain. To go and look for "evidence" of agency outside the domain of storytelling seems to imply the opposite: that storytelling and agency are essentially separated; that storytelling happens in one place, and agency can be affected or not by it, in a different life context.

What is more, as I explained in the introduction, to try to obtain ethnographic data from patients' daily lives is highly problematic from a reflexive, feminist ethical standpoint to which the current study subscribes.

So this book relies on the accounts patients produce: the e-mail and face-to-face accounts patients gave me as a researcher, and the accounts they give to each other online. Both situations—the act of constructing an account and telling it to the researcher (a stranger), and engaging in storytelling online—are considered as part of the wider ongoing process in which patients construct their self-narratives. Through these different situations I could access patients' storytelling. By drawing on patients' accounts of their online experience, I introduce the possibility of thinking about storytelling as a process that has the potential to interweave their online and offline worlds.

CHAPTER 3

Storytelling and Therapy in the Context of Breast Cancer and Chronic Illness

Participants' online activities do not take place in a vacuum. In Chapter 2 I discussed the limitation of thinking about the online space and participants' experiences as an isolated social phenomenon. To understand why and how breast cancer patients engage in online spaces to communicate their illness and produce their stories, we must look beyond what is going on online. As Jones (2004, p. 326) commented, "The things we do by using the internet today are in need of both radical contextualization and radical historicization." Indeed, to adequately account for what breast cancer patients do online, we need to contextualize their experience, and locate it historically, a task that involves exploring the broader cultural and communicative environment within which patients' online activity is embedded. The communicative environment, in turn, is being shaped and transformed through patients' online engagement.

This chapter focuses on the cultural and communicative context that frames, shapes and is shaped by patients' storytelling online. More specifically, the discussion explores the key underlying discourses and cultural themes that constitute this communicative context. The focus is on the culture of breast cancer in contemporary society, and how it is interlinked with discourses of chronic illness and therapy. The discussion shows how storytelling and narrative have become central in the social and cultural construction of breast cancer and its therapeutic discourse. It provides the backdrop for understanding breast cancer patients' storytelling online, as explored in later chapters.

The Place of Breast Cancer in Contemporary Culture: Historical Perspective

> Today breast cancer is the biggest disease on the cultural map—bigger than AIDS, cystic fibrosis or spinal injury. It is bigger even than those more prolific killers of women—heart diseases, lung cancer and stroke. There are hundreds of web-sites devoted to it, not to mention newsletters, support groups, a whole genre of first-person breast cancer books; even, in the US, a glossy, upper-middle brow, monthly magazine. There are pink ribbon days and an annual "race for the cure" in the US which attracts a million people. (Ehrenreich, 2001, p. 1a)

Breast cancer has an extremely visible and voluble presence in contemporary culture. Notably, for instance, there has been overcoverage of breast cancer in the media, compared to incidence of the disease in the population (Saywell, Henderson, and Beattie, 2000; Seale, 2001). The preoccupation of contemporary culture with aspects of embodied femininity, particularly the breast, has inevitably resulted in breast cancer "taking residence in every cultural medium, from soap operas to sculpture" and so "There is no public forum now in which breast cancer is not at home" (Leopold, 1999, p. 2).

However, breast cancer came to prominence quite recently. During the nineteenth century, and through the first half of the twentieth century, it was completely cordoned off from the public arena. It was "a private experience suffered by women individually, at the margins of public consciousness" (p. 3). Like cancer in general, and any other taboo subject, breast cancer had to be hidden away from public view. The disfigurement it brought was thought to be a precursor of certain death. Unlike other deformities such as the effects of leprosy, however, signs of breast cancer could be hidden away. Thus, a woman who suffered with breast cancer was encouraged to disguise her pain and discomfort not only to the outside world but also to herself (p. 204). As a consequence, "virtually no woman with breast cancer was aware of anyone else suffering with it. And the language that would have enabled her to discuss her condition with a fellow sufferer, to exchange, for instance, information about symptoms and the side effects of treatment, was not available to her" (p. 204). In short, during the nineteenth century and the beginning of the twentieth century, there was no infrastructure for women to communicate the disease (p. 213).

A gradual change started to take place by the turn of the century, especially with the increasing availability of surgery and the introduction of the radical mastectomy as the "gold standard" (that is, the dominant model of treatment for breast cancer; p. 10). In the late 1930s, first-person cancer narratives written by women began to appear in popular magazines, starting to switch the perspective from the impersonal medical (predominantly male) authority voice, to the more intimate voice of personal experience. Those early stories, however, kept portraying the doctor as the main, if not the exclusive, source of information and knowledge that a woman has (p. 219). Consequently, the knowledge that women had was of a "need-to-know" nature, with doctors conveying just enough knowledge to gain the women's cooperation while sustaining their status as patients rather than as partners (p. 183). So despite these changes, women's experience of the disease remained largely sealed off from the public arena.

The first meaningful landmark in the assimilation of women into the communication of the disease was the foundation of the Women's Field Army (WFA) in 1936, by the American Society for Cancer Control (ASCC). The WFA was an explicit attempt to challenge the passivity towards breast cancer and the fatalism that dominated both medical and public attitudes towards the disease. By raising public awareness about breast cancer and its curability, the WFA sought to fight the continued silence and stigma that surrounded the disease (Lerner, 2001, p. 43). Yet despite the support garnered by the WFA, by the mid 1960s, the number of American women dying from breast cancer every year had surpassed 25,000 and seemed to be rising. Despite the large number, women had no idea of how large a sorority they belonged to (Leopold, 1999, p. 153).

It was not until the early 1970s that the illness significantly emerged within the public cultural arena. A significant contribution to the "coming out" of the illness "from the closet to the commonplace" (p. 215) was the publication of patients' personal stories in the mass media. Highly prominent among those stories was *Why Me?* (Kushner, 1977), an account written by Rose Kushner, a Baltimore journalist diagnosed in 1974, who turned her breast cancer into a public crusade to inform women about the disease and their treatment options. A subsequent contribution to the opening up of the discussion on the illness was *First, You Cry* (Rollin, 1976), a vivid account by Betty Rollin, an NBC correspondent, of her experience with breast cancer (Lerner, 2001, p. xii). Perhaps most influential, however, were famous American women such as Shirley Temple Black, Betty Ford, and Happy Rockefeller who, during the 1970s, revealed their diagnoses in the media (p. 7). "The press served as a critical intermediary between the closed world of medical science on the one hand and the equally sequestered world of breast cancer patients it was deemed to serve on the other" (Leopold, 1999, p. 231).

Television also played a central role in bringing the disease into the open. Highly significant was the first televised portrayal of breast cancer in the soap opera *The Young and the Restless* (broadcast in 1974), giving rise to many more occasions for breast cancer to appear on television and be incorporated into many dramatic series (p. 241). Particularly pertinent to the current discussion is the focus that representation of breast cancer on television gave to the personal experience of the illness and its reinforcement of breast cancer as a personal story. The increasing availability of patients' personal stories significantly contributed to the raising of the visibility of the illness and the opening up of its discussion. This background is important to the discussion in later chapters of the availability and centrality of storytelling in contemporary online environments of breast cancer patients. Also vital is an understanding of the dominant meanings of breast cancer, a topic that I take up in the next section.

Dominant Meanings of Breast Cancer

Alternative or competing voices to the dominant meanings of breast cancer remain largely in the margins of the breast cancer debate. While alternative kinds of narrative do emerge, for example, ones that explicitly state they do not want to speak of bravery and courage in fighting the disease, these voices are still contained; and even within these voices, the notion of the courageous fighter comes through "the back door" in more implicit ways (Potts, 2000, p. 111). I therefore do not explore those meanings in this chapter. I do, however, in relevant places in the analysis of the online communication of breast cancer, consider the extent to which competing messages to the dominant ones are being voiced. Generally speaking, while the online environment is often celebrated as a discursive space that allows for alternative (even radical) messages to dominant discourses to be communicated, I remain unconvinced of this claim in the context of breast cancer.

Self-responsibility. Since their early days in the 1920s, breast cancer public education campaigns conditioned women to accept responsibility for whatever calamities befell them (Leopold, 1999, p. 161). With the focus on the illness as a private experience on an intimate scale, women were encouraged to look inward rather than outward (p. 184). As with the campaign against cervical cancer, so too with breast cancer; the 1950s seemed to have been an even riper time to promote the message of patients' self-responsibility: "Having emerged from the Depression, defeated the Germans and Japanese in World War II, undergone an economic boom, and invested in scientific research, the United States suddenly seemed within reach of making cervical cancer a curable disease" (Lerner, 2001, p. 51).

A particularly common approach in the 1950s was to tell the story of a woman whose recent death had resulted from her unwillingness to participate in breast cancer detection strategies. Thus the line between responsibility and blame was extremely thin (p. 59), and the relationship between the two was encapsulated in the form of a personal story. Later, as the techniques grew more sophisticated, moving from breast self-examinations to screening mammography, the survival rates did improve but the underlying strategy remained unchanged: the emphasis on early detection shifted attention and accountability away from the medical profession and towards the patient and her personal behavior (Leopold, 1999, p. 174).

The emphasis on women's responsibility for their own cure has had a huge impact on the discourse of breast cancer that continues even today. For example, a recent study (Charles, Whelan, Gafni, Reyno and Redko, 1998) has shown that the governing construction of treatment decision making among breast cancer patients is that "doing nothing is no choice." Patients internalize the idea that they are responsible for their treatment and cure: they have to constantly reassure themselves that they have done everything possible to maximize their treatment (and thus their healing) options.

Leopold (1999) describes this bias towards self-responsibility as part of the "privatization" of breast cancer. The open recognition of the disease, argues Leopold, has not been accompanied by the emergence of any sense of social responsibility. The stress has been increasingly on the intimate, individual struggle between the disease and its victim, with a focus on breast cancer being predominantly a domestic drama.

The message of personal responsibility and enhanced involvement of the patient implies, among other things, a shift in the control of the communicative space of the disease, primarily from the hands of the medical profession to those of the laypersons. One of the consequences of this shift is that embodied knowledge often turns out to be more reliable than biomedical knowledge, particularly for women who experienced technological or biomedical failures such as detection failures (Fosket, 2000). This shift is a significant context for the emergence of the Internet as "patients' queendom," as I describe it in Chapter 4—that is, as a communicative space that legitimizes, values and foregrounds patients' experiential and embodied knowledge, especially in the form of storytelling.

Triumphalism, cheerfulness, hope and survival

> In the seamless world of breast cancer culture, where one website links to another—from personal narratives and grassroots endeavours to the glitzy level of corporate sponsors and celebrity spokespeople—cheerfulness is more or less mandatory, dissent a kind of treason. (Ehrenreich, 2001, p. 1a)

> Breast cancer talk on the Internet is a self-directed rhetoric of hope and enablement.... [I]ts many threads form a blanket of nurturance that helps to promote the transformation of vulnerability into strength, and negativity into hopefulness. (Sharf, 1997, p. 78)

As both quotes usefully observe, the discourse of breast cancer (in its offline and online manifestations) is clearly governed by optimism. Self-help and personal responsibility are constructed as key to hope and enablement. The following extract from one of my interviewees' online accounts is testimony to this utopian claim:

> I was diagnosed on 7/8/99 with invasive lobular breast cancer. It took a couple of days for the news to "sink in" and then I felt I had a choice. I could be a "victim" of this disease ... or I could face it head on ~ with a positive attitude and *"just do it."* I chose to be bigger than the cancer and face it head on. (E-mail 14 [italics added])

It should be said, however, that the motifs of hope and the "triumphalism of survivorhood," as somewhat cynically described by Ehrenreich (2001, p. 1a), are not unique to the discourse of breast cancer, but are characteristic of the wider discourse of cancer. Stacey (1997), for instance, has shown how the dominant cancer narrative, evident in a number of different genres (popular culture, medical, feminist), is one of heroism, of confronting the monsters, battling against the odds, and of triumph. Sontag's well-known analysis of *Illness as Metaphor* (1978) also accounts for the "triumphal" dimension as constitutive of the construction of cancer. She fascinatingly demonstrates this point by reflecting on the association of the cancer personality with one of life's losers (p. 48). In the case of breast cancer, claims Potts (2000, p. 111), this triumphalism often takes the form of "a trajectory in which the heroine emerges richer for her experience, a 'better person,' the kind of woman we are all supposed to be, who copes with whatever life throws at her." Patients' online stories, as I will show throughout the analysis, often answer to this description.

One of the implications of a discourse governed by such notions is the almost complete exclusion of death from the discussion. It appears as if, in the culture of breast cancer, death is a taboo: "Why is there no room in this cult for some gracious acceptance of death, when the time comes, which it surely will, through cancer or other misfortune?" (Ehrenreich, 2001, p. 1a). Sharf's (1997) analysis of the online communication of a breast cancer mailing list bears out this observation: "Participants have decided to emphasize hope, tempered by realism, and to make this a colloquy about living with breast cancer, rather than dying from it" (p. 73).

Another aspect tied in with the governance of hope of the discourse of breast cancer is the construction of the illness as a site of continuous change, rather than as a fixed, determined experience. It is only by regarding the illness experience as constantly and dynamically changing that hope and cheerfulness can have meaningful room in its representation. The introduction to *Dr. Susan Love's Breast Book* (Love, 2000), a breast cancer guide often referred to by patients as the "bible of breast cancer," neatly demonstrates this idea in describing the study of the breast as a "work-in-progress" (Love, 2000, p. xvii).

Love's account, a primary text in the discourse of breast cancer, epitomizes the dominant way in which the scene of breast cancer is portrayed in the public discourse: dynamic and ever changing. By the same token, a common metaphor used to describe one's experience with breast cancer (and cancer in general) is that of a "journey" (e.g., McLellan, 1997), implying movement and change rather than fixity and fatalism. One can already think about the role online communication could potentially play in this scene, for its immediate and dynamic character.

Military discourse and the language of warfare. Hand in glove with optimism and triumphalism goes the language of warfare and struggle. In the years after World War II, to motivate American women to participate in the effort of early detection of breast cancer, combat metaphors were used, linking the "war" on breast cancer with recent American military triumphs. For instance, the cover of the Women's Field Army pamphlet showed a picture of a sword, titled as the "Sword of Hope." Even more obvious is the very choice to form a body of women volunteers, under the name of "Women's Field Army."

The language of war is characteristic not only of the discourse of breast cancer, but of cancer in general. Sontag's seminal work (1978) provides a thoughtful analysis of the prevalence of warfare language in the construction of cancer in our culture. Cancer, argues Sontag, fills the role of an illness experienced as ruthless, secret invasion (p. 5). It is commonly described as a process in which the body is consumed (p. 10), "invaded" by alien cells (p. 13), and "with the patient's body considered to be under attack ('invasion'), the only treatment is counterattack" (p. 63). The treatment is also described by military rhetoric. It aims to kill cancer cells and the fight against cancer often sounds like a colonial war (p. 65). Seale (2001) too, in a recent account of the predominance of sporting language in news reports of cancer experience, reflects on the domination of military connotations in current representations of cancer.

Contextualizing the Dominant Meanings of Breast Cancer

So far I have focused on the social and cultural construction of breast cancer from a historical perspective. I discussed the dominant meanings that emerged from this construction, and highlighted the centrality of storytelling and patients' personal narratives in the circulation and perpetuation of those meanings. Next, I locate these meanings within three broader contexts, which are inextricably tied in to the culture of breast cancer and its communication. These contexts provide an interesting and necessary background for the discussion in later chapters of what breast cancer patients do online, particularly their engagement in storytelling.

The American Context

As we have seen, the discourse of breast cancer is clearly one of personal responsibility, imbued with the ideology of self-help and the language of war. Although these discursive elements are universal characteristics of the culture of breast cancer, they have a significant American imprint. First, the historical and cultural context in which breast cancer emerged is American. While other Western countries had established cancer control by the 1930s, the emphasis on mobilizing the public against the cancer nemesis was most pronounced in the United States, with its rich historical legacy of citizens forming interest groups in order to promote social reform. Anticancer organizations outside the United States (England's Imperial Cancer Research Institute, for example) tended to focus more on promoting research than waging a war of propaganda against the disease. "Europeans" stated the director of the American Society for Cancer Control in 1939, "have toward the cancer problem a much more patient, long-time attitude than we do in America" (cited in Lerner, 2001, p. 45).

Second, as Leopold (1999, pp. 172–173) observes, the insistence on personal responsibility that dominates so many aspects of American life has a clear part in this construction. In this context, Albom (1998, p. 65) describes America as "a Persian bazaar of self-help." In a culture that has always valued the virtues of self-help, says Leopold, one finds it hard to escape the self-blame that accompanies failure. A belief in self-determination and autonomy has always been part of the ideology of the United States, following Benjamin Franklin's notion of autonomous self-help, that is, the idea that "one could help oneself" to shape a life uniquely satisfying and unfettered (Grodin and Lindlof, 1996, p. 5). The discourses of breast cancer work by the same cultural rationale: to internalize the problem and to search for its remedy within one's body.

Third, the language of war has significant American resonance. As also evidenced by the "war on poverty," the "war on drugs," and more recently the "war on terror," Americans often characterize efforts to combat social problems in terms of battle.

This cultural bias of breast cancer culture and discourse has important consequences for the character of breast cancer online spaces. In the following chapters I show that any attempt to explain the social significance of breast cancer patients' online communication must account for the cultural American context in which it is embedded. I demonstrate how what breast cancer patients do online, especially their engagement in storytelling, is fundamentally demarcated by North American linguistic, national, temporal, spatial, religious, ideological and discursive borders.

The Ethical Context of the Enterprising Self

The message of personal responsibility and self-help is embedded in a cultural ethical regime that is governed by ideas of "survivalism" (Lasch, 1980), the "autonomization," "responsibilization" (Rose, 1992) and the "individualization of the self" (Beck, 2001). Although each of these notions has particular meanings and implications, and despite some significant differences between them, they all enlighten the idea that contemporary everyday life has been increasingly patterned by techniques of self-management and self-steering. In the cultural ethical regime of the "enterprising self" (Rose, 1992) people no longer perceive themselves as subjects with duties and obligations, but as individuals with rights and freedoms, with the powers of personal choice, self-fulfillment and initiative (Beck, 2001; Rose, 1992).

A key site where the vocabulary and discourse of the self are exercised and constructed is health. Patients are depicted as "health workers" (Stacey, 1988), actively seeking to understand and make sense of their illness and treatments (Lambert and Rose, 1996). This depiction has had great resonance in the recent debate on "e-patients." The latter are seen as active consumers of health information and creative producers of lay knowledge. In this construction, the Internet is seen as empowering patients in providing them with tools to fulfill their role as "health consumers" (e.g., Hardey, 2001). This is an important context for understanding breast cancer patients' active involvement in online spaces, particularly in the construction of their self-narratives online. However, my account discusses this phenomenon more critically. That is, the discussion does not just celebrate the Internet as a space that "empowers" patients by allowing them the means and the space to fulfill themselves as "health workers" and exercise their "autonomous self," but also considers the more critical consequences of the phenomenon. In particular, it questions how a communicative space where patients' stories of their experience focus on their self-responsibility contributes to the broader increasing shift of responsibilities from society to individuals, and especially from the health system to patients (Leopold, 1999).[11]

The Feminist Context

A third significant context within which the dominant representations of breast cancer are embedded is the feminist debate (Potts, 2000).

Cancer in general has been seen historically as a "female disease": "Women have long been taught that cancer is their special concern and that, indeed, to worry about cancer is their duty" (Reagan, 1997, cited in Lerner, 2001, p. 46). The language of war on cancer, and on breast cancer in particular, was often linked specifically to women: "It was a women's war," noted a WFA pamphlet, "because they have the patience, devotion, and the courage needed" (Lerner, 2001, p. 46, citing a WFA pamphlet).

The decision to designate women as "volunteer soldiers" for the WFA in the 1930s did not necessarily have to do with the high prevalence of the disease,[12] but with women being relegated to the private sphere of the home and their citizenship being tied into the production of other healthy citizens, that is, their families, their communities, and so on (Lerner, 2001, p. 46). Interestingly, the recent figures on women being the main seekers of health information online are consistent with this construction. Women appear to go online not only for their own health-related issues, but also as caregivers to family members and friends (Pew Internet & American Life, 2002b).

Despite the explicit connection between women and breast cancer, the disease entered the public debate as part of the women's health movement only in the 1990s (Leopold, 1999, pp. 190–191). This delayed response enabled breast cancer to exploit the feminist principles that early women's health movements' campaigns brought into the public arena and legitimized, namely the idea that women have "the right to choose" and to determine the outcomes that might affect their own health (p. 194). So the communication of issues such as abortion during the 1960s and the 1970s paved the way for breast cancer's projection into public debate. Eventually breast cancer became meaningfully implicated in the feminist project of the women's health movement in the 1970s and the 1980s. It was part of the movement's effort to expose the "socially constructed and punishable shamefulness of all aspects of female embodiment" (Potts, 2000, p. 99).

One of the manifestations of this tenet has been the emphasis on women's writing as a central means for the creation of sisterhood and camaraderie. Feminist discourse has long underscored the public and political significance of women writing their lives, "taking the power of words, of representation, into their own hands" (Friedman, 1988, p. 40). Indeed, in the context of breast cancer, writers of their own personal accounts often describe their search for other women who had

had breast cancer and who could help them in their own understanding of the illness (Potts, 2000). The prominence of patients' engagement in storytelling online—which I discuss in later chapters—cannot be fully understood without this context of the centrality of writing as a political activity in the feminist project.

Therapy and Storytelling

The production of selfhood as a project of self-transformation and development has particular resonance in relation to the feminine subject (Blackman, 2004, p. 232). However, beyond the feminist agenda, contemporary culture is increasingly characterized by the flourishing of different culturally mediated forms of disclosure, confession and self-revelation. Media forms such as television talk shows, advice books or popular magazines are central sites for the proliferation of discourses of confession and therapy (Blackman, 2004; Peck, 1996; White, 1992). Individuals, female audiences in particular, are encouraged to work on themselves through particular techniques of self-production and self-help. One of the key therapeutic techniques available in, and promoted by, contemporary media spaces is talking and writing the self—and more specifically, storytelling.

In what follows I develop this discussion, to highlight writing and storytelling as part of the broader therapeutic model that pervades contemporary culture, particularly in the context of chronic illness. In profound ways, this model backs up, legitimizes and shapes what breast cancer patients do online.

The Therapeutic in the "Talking Cure"

The therapeutic model of storytelling is rooted in the psychoanalytical notion of the "talking cure." Since Freud's inauguration of psychoanalysis, the reconstruction of a coherent self-narrative has been held as a therapeutic goal (Polkinghorne, 1991, p. 150). A recent interest in the processual and hermeneutic nature of psychotherapeutic practices (Mattingly and Garro, 2000, p. 7) has brought forward the argument about the significance of narrative construction for the process of therapeutic change.

Brooks' account in *Psychoanalysis and Storytelling* (1994) is a pertinent point of reference in this discussion. In it, Brooks emphasizes storytelling as a means of establishing "truth." He argues that the work of narrative construction is a process that aims at finding an explanation that will resume in the future towards a desired end. Storytelling is geared towards finding a workable "truth." Spence (1982) termed it "narrative truth":

> [W]hat we have in mind when we say that such and such is a good story, that a given explanation carries conviction, that *one* solution to a mystery must be true. Once a given construction has acquired narrative truth, it becomes just as real as any kind of truth; this new reality becomes a significant part of the psychoanalytic cure. (p. 31, italics in original)

A well-constructed and coherent narrative possesses a kind of narrative truth that is "real and immediate and carries an important significance for the process of therapeutic change" (Spence, 1982, p. 21). In other words, the work of storytelling is seen as the fundamental process in seeking and achieving a cure. It enables and strengthens the capacity of the storyteller (in the psychoanalytical context, the analysand) to contextualize things that are beyond his/her control.

Fundamentally, in assuming psychoanalysis as the scene of storytelling, theorists (Brooks, 1994; Schafer, 1980; Spence, 1982) accentuate the source of therapy in the process of making a story, rather than in the actual story that is being produced. Ogden (2000) summarizes this idea in his discussion of the process of mourning following emotional losses: "What one 'makes' in the process of mourning ... is far less important than the experience of making it" (p. 66).

Storytelling and Illness

The therapeutic model of storytelling has become increasingly central in the discussion on patients' coping with illness (particularly chronic illness), among both social researchers of health and illness and medical professionals. The growing theoretical importance of the narrative concept in the field of illness research reflects the increasing emphasis on suffering as a point of departure for the study of illness (Hydén, 1997, p. 52) and the increasing focus in medical sociology upon people's subjective experiences in the contexts of their daily lives, their culture and their biographies (Bury, 1982; Lawton, 2003; Radley, 1993; Williams, 1984).

Within medical anthropology and the sociology of health and illness, narrative and storytelling are commonly seen as a means of conveying the biographical disruption caused by illness, especially chronic illness (Bury, 1982; Frank, 1995; Kleinman, 1988; Mattingly and Garro, 2000).[13] Accounts such as *The Wounded Storyteller* (Frank, 1995), *The Illness Narratives* (Kleinman, 1988), and *The Cancer Journals* (Lorde, 1980) highlight illness as "a call for stories" (Frank, 1995, p. 53): a situation of crisis that invigorates a creative engagement in an interpretative activity of constructing a story.

The point of departure for understanding the significance and centrality of storytelling for patients' coping is the notion of disruption. Illness, chronic illness in particular, constitutes a disruption or a disturbance of the continuity of people's everyday life (Bury, 1982). Bury framed this aspect as "biographical disruption" to highlight the way in which acute illness alters the relationship between the patient's body, self and surrounding environment.

As a consequence of this disruption, patients engage in what Frank (1995, p. 54) describes as "a repair work on the wreck": a continuous endeavor to manage this disturbance by regaining their ontological security and the continuity of their self-identity, fundamentals that have been seriously threatened. In this context, storytelling plays a central role in patients' coping (Bury, 1982, 1991; Becker, 1994; Hydén, 1997, p. 51; Williams, 1984). The notion of narrative reconstruction describes the conceptual strategies people employ to create a sense of coherence, stability, control and order in the aftermath of the "biographically disruptive" event of illness (Lawton, 2003, p. 27). Storytelling is seen as enabling the storyteller to regain order and reestablish continuity in life after a disruption. It provides an arena for coming to terms with a problematic experience and making sense of what is happening. Through stories, patients convey how the lived experience of chronic pain affects the way they thought about themselves, their lives and their futures (Mattingly and Garro, 2000, p. 28).

Medical sociologists and anthropologists regard storytelling as a way of contextualizing illness events, experiences and symptoms, by weaving them together within a biographical context. Storytelling enables patients to give meanings to events that have disrupted and altered the course of their lives (Bury, 1991; Hydén, 1997, p. 51; Williams, 1984). In this context, Frank (1985) highlights the process of storytelling as an exercise by which ill people refuse their bodies' surrender to illness and medicine, reclaiming their control over their bodies and their capacity to act.

In short, storytelling is a way for a patient who has suffered a severe crisis in life to come through it, emerging as a new or regenerated human being (Hydén, 1997). The act of writing is seen as a crucial affirmation of living, a statement against fearfulness, invisibility and silence (Lorde, 1980, p. 61). It is a way to give meaning against the meaninglessness of the disease experience (Acker, 1997). Thus, the construction of narrative is one way of becoming capable of thinking beyond the constraints of one's conditions, to realize one's transformative capacity.

As far as medical practice is concerned, recently there has been growing recognition of the role that storytelling can play in helping patients cope with their illness (e.g., Calman, 2001; Carlick and Biley, 2004; Heiney, 1995). The use of creative and expressive arts in cancer care—writing and storytelling being one of them—has been increasingly recognized as a vehicle through which patients can find meaning in their illness and move into a new life beyond cancer (Carlick and Biley, 2004; Ferris and Stein, 2002). Carlick and Biley (2004) urge oncology nurses to integrate the use of narratives into their practice and raise awareness among professionals of the therapeutic potential of storytelling. This, they argue, will not only enable cancer patients to develop coping skills, but will also assist in the progression and improvement of twenty-first-century health care practice. They view the incorporation of the therapeutic storytelling model into the practice of medical professionals as a way to return to the "art of caring," which they consider an essential complement to "the science of curing" (pp. 314–315, drawing on Watson, 1985, 1999).

The medical profession has only quite recently started exploring the potential role that the Internet may play in this context. Two examples from the United Kingdom are DIPEx and the Expert Patient Programme (Carlick and Biley, 2004, p. 315). DIPEx is a charity funded by a variety of health care sources, including the U.K. Department of Health. It runs a website[14] where patients are invited to share their personal experiences of health and illness. Patients' stories on a variety of health contexts can be read (as texts), listened to (as audio files only) or viewed (as audiovisual files). DIPEx's broader effort is to collect illness narratives in a systematic fashion from patients with a wide range of conditions and treatments, "in order to ground patient information, professional education and research in the illness experience" (Yaphe, Rigge, Herxheimer, McPherson, Miller, Shepperd, and Ziebland, 2000, p. 180). The Expert Patients Programme[15] is a U.K. National Health

Service (NHS) based training program that aims at providing people who live with long-term chronic illness with skills to manage their condition better on a day-to-day basis. As part of this goal, the program uses its website to display patients' narratives.

Despite evidence of this kind, it still seems quite difficult to ascertain the degree to which medical professionals accept and encourage patients to engage in storytelling online. The available data seems to relate mainly to health professionals' attitudes towards patients' use of the Internet for information seeking, rather than for therapeutic storytelling. Even within this body of research, there seem to be contradictory findings. Some argue that health professionals welcome patients' information seeking on the Internet, while others indicate that health professionals are not comfortable with their patients' growing involvement in information seeking online (Cox, 2002; Dolan, 2003). Clearly, as I mentioned in Chapter 2, information seeking has been the paradigm that governed the way in which patients' use of the Internet has been understood till now. It would be interesting and potentially fruitful to learn more about the medical profession's approach to patients' engagement in storytelling online, and the degree to which this model is encouraged, if at all.

To summarize, the intention of this chapter has been to identify the underlying cultural ideas and meanings of breast cancer and their relation to broader discourses of chronic illness, therapy and storytelling. Shedding light on the cultural communicative environment of breast cancer is essential for understanding the significance and the consequences of online communication for women who suffer from the disease in the twenty-first century. Given the historical context of the silencing of breast cancer and its very recent unveiling, the question of the role played by patients' online communication of the disease and patients' participation in telling their stories online seems ever more salient. What kind of communicative infrastructure does the online environment furnish to patients today? What makes the online environment so attractive to them? Why does online communication fit so well with the broader communicative environment of the disease? In what ways do online spaces enable patients to engage in therapeutic storytelling and what are the consequences of this practice for their lives? These questions are explored in the coming chapters.

CHAPTER 4

Emplotment and the Construction of Closure

I don't know how many people search for "cancer *experience*" but it's more likely they'd search for "cancer story." (E, the designer of a cancer patients' website, interview 5)

For E, a cancer website designer, that patients search for illness stories online seems commonsensical. Yet, as I discussed in earlier chapters, participants' storytelling online has been largely overlooked and not studied much. When it comes to patients, the focus has been mainly on their engagement in information seeking online, experience exchange and self-presentation, but there has been very little research on the aspect of storytelling.

This chapter aims to account for the centrality of the processes and forms of storytelling that emerge in patients' online communication of breast cancer. My point of departure for this exploration is the notion of storytelling as introduced in Chapter 2. I start by examining how patients' online experiences facilitate the production of their self-narratives: "constellations of *relationships* (connected parts) embedded in *time and space*, constituted by *causal emplotment*" (Somers, 1994, p. 616, italics in original). In light of this definition, I explore how a process of emplotment takes place in online spaces, how elements of one's experience are being configured into a whole on online sites, and how processes of online communication work to direct them towards closure.

Unlike other authors who studied online illness narratives (Hardey, 2001, 2002; McLellan, 1997), I do not pursue a consistent comparison between online and traditional illness narratives. Thinking about online narratives only in relational terms, that is, against conventional offline narratives, reproduces the conceptual and methodological separation between the online and the offline. It also constrains our ability to recognize the potential distinctive qualities of storytelling online that are not necessarily comparable to other modes of storytelling.

My intention is to appraise what is significant and perhaps distinctive about the process of storytelling when it takes place online. I start by discussing patients' need to make sense. This is the primary condition for their decision to engage in storytelling online. I then explore how the online communicative environment of breast cancer furnishes patients with frameworks of meaning for the construction of their stories. Next, I examine how patients' online experience directs them towards a construction of closure. As I discussed in Chapter 2, one of the key features that characterizes the process of storytelling and distinguishes it from other communicative processes is the imposition of, or the attempt to impose, closure on the account of events. I describe patients' struggle to construct closure as a dialectical process that entails remembering the painful experience and at the same time insists on a closure of the painful chapter and moving on towards an optimistic future. In particular, I examine the inextricable link between storytelling and survival, and its significance in patients' online communication. Finally, I explore situations in which patients stop engaging in storytelling online. Looking at why patients stop engaging in this interpretative work enlightens our understanding of the meaning of the actual act of storytelling online, and helps to further clarify its scope and limits. I conclude by integrating the different aspects discussed in the chapter into an argument about the role of storytelling online and its consequences.

The Quest for Making Sense

A Fragmented Reality, a Fragmented Representation

I would like to open the discussion of this issue with two extracts from patients' accounts. The first excerpt is the opening paragraph of an e-mail account of a 51-year-old breast cancer survivor (whom I refer to as B), who relates her online experience in the context of her illness. The second excerpt is part of a face-to-face interview with J, a 44-year-old breast cancer survivor.

(1)

I was Dx 10/98 - I found the lump in my breast; mammography failed to detect it. Ultrasound with guide wire confirmed lump. Lumpectomy 11/98 - results invasive ductal carcinoma and DCIS (ductal carcinoma in tisu) -pre-cancerous cells. Lumpectomy did not achieve "clean margins"-when they slice the tumour for pathology they ink the edges. If edges are "clean" they have gotten all the cancer. 11/98 had a wide excision (large lumpectomy) and axillary dissection (lymph node removal). No positive nodes (good sign that cancer has not spread further than the breast) but unclean margins again. 12/98 had mastectomy. (E-mail 2)

(2)
Q: *What kinds of things were you looking for (when you went online)?*
J: I wanted to know, really: Me! (laughs). 43 old male, oh female! pre-menopausal, has this kind of cancer, at this stage, several lymph nodes, what's going to happen? And of course, I was probably looking for the impossible. (J, interview 10)

It is clear from both excerpts that the diagnosis is the background for the online experience; this is what frames patients' motivation to go online. In the first excerpt, B starts her account with a detailed report of her diagnosis. The different elements of her diagnosis constitute the backdrop for her engagement online. Similarly, in the second excerpt, J describes her expectations from the Internet as deriving directly from the specific elements of her diagnosis.

B's and J's accounts, as well as accounts of other interviewees, describe the diagnosis in a very fragmented way. The diagnosis appears as a set of terms and elements that are totally foreign to the patient's life, lacking any meaningful connection between them. Had B's account not been written in the first person, one could have easily thought it were part of a laboratory medical report; the language is highly medical and the style extremely informative, laconic and impersonal. By the same token, J's description of her diagnosis constitutes a set of elements that appear totally disjointed: 43-year-old female/premenopausal/breast cancer/stage X/several lymph nodes. This kind of representation resembles what Hayden White, in his seminal essay "The Value of Narrativity in the Representation of Reality" (1980), referred to as annals. This form of representation "possesses none of the attributes that we normally think of as a story: no central subject, no well-marked beginning, middle, and end, no peripeteia, and no identifiable narrative voice" (p. 7). It does not suggest any necessary connection between one element and another, and all elements seem to have the same order of importance or unimportance. Finally, it "does not conclude; it simply terminates" (p. 8).

However, unlike the historian annalist,[16] for a breast cancer patient it is impossible to sustain her experience in such a disjointed form. To manage the disturbance posed by the cancer to the "normality" of her everyday life, she seeks to connect the fragmented elements of her diagnosis into a coherent and plausible framework. Narrative provides this framework: it is geared towards making sense of her experience. It aims to direct the seemingly unconnected elements towards a closure; as J puts it, "What's going to happen to me?" It enables participants to emplot their experience and direct it towards a certain closure. In what follows, I account for the ways in which this process works online.

Going Online as a Means of Dissipating "the Fog of Confusion and Fear"

> I have found the internet to be extremely useful and have found several sites ... that have helped me through the fog of confusion and fear. (A message posted by a breast cancer patient on a message board)

The quest for sense making is a central factor in women's motivation to go online in the context of their illness. Interviewees' descriptions of the situation that prefaced their referral to the Internet portray a fairly chaotic state of mind, in which they had many questions and unknown fears. Indicative of this total confusion is J's experience (interview 10). Despite her familiarity with the illness (both her mother and grandmother suffered from breast cancer) when she first went online to search for information about the disease, she had to find out how to spell "breast cancer." The following online account is another testimony of the uncertainty that governs patients' condition following the diagnosis of breast cancer (note the repetitive use of ellipsis points, indicating confusion and uncertainty):

> Everyone is afraid and wants to know what the other has gone thru what they should do ... where they can get information, so they can make the right choices for them ... what to ask their doctors ... how to be their own advocate ... how to deal with side effects, and what side effects to expect? How are we dealing with the trama of losing our hair and being bald.... Our families, relations with our spouses, our children, friends, our jobs, insurance, indifferent doctors, or bosses.... Depression, fatigue..., where to find local support..., dealing with the loss of their breast/breasts ... to reconstruct or not?... there are million questions. (E-mail 15)

The diagnosis is perhaps the stage where confusion and uncertainty are most acute, as was shown in the accounts of B and J. Unsurprisingly, it is often the time when women refer to the Internet and start engaging in an attempt to make sense of their situation. However, confusion and uncertainty are lurking features of the experience of the illness, especially since the reality of breast cancer does not allow final closure—there is always the risk of recurrence. Therefore, the project of "making sense," particularly through storytelling, is a work in progress. It helps patients to configure elements into a whole by "grasping them together," directing them toward a conclusion or ending (Polkinghorne, 1991, p. 141).

Frameworks of Meaning for Storytelling Online

The online experience furnishes patients with available frameworks of meaning with which they can organize and make sense of their experience. These frameworks are constituted by other women's stories and by the visual and textual manners in which breast cancer websites are structured. These frameworks are characterized by four key principles: (1) locating experience in time and space; (2) "gluing" together of elements by an overriding topic; (3) providing an asynchronous environment as a framework for storytelling; and (4) establishing the authority of a storyteller. In what follows, I demonstrate how these principles facilitate patients' storytelling online.

Locating experience in time and space

> Let's try and organize the thoughts ... chronologically it's probably the easiest thing, isn't it? It's an easy structure to work with. (K, interview 11)

I think that it is not accidental that the above quote is the way in which K started her account in her interview. Breast cancer patients look for an "easy structure to work with," to organize their experience within a coherent framework that they can inspect, think about and plan actions around. As K suggests, one element that may provide this "easy structure" is a chronological ordering of the experience of the illness. A visit to various breast cancer websites in which patients publish the stories of their illness reveals how, through narratives, participants order different events by linking them together within a broader sequential framework. Hardey (2002) makes a similar observation in his study of home pages of people's illnesses. However, beyond the fact that these stories are performed in the online space, there is nothing new in arguing that the narrative orders the experience in time and space. At stake is the question of the specificity of the online communication in enabling this ordering of experience in space and time. What is it in the online environment that facilitates the construction of an "easy structure to work with"?

"Shared Experience" website[17] is a useful example to start addressing this question. It is defined as a "Cancer Support Knowledgebase," designed to enable cancer patients and their caregivers to share their experience of illness online.

Figure 3 *"Shared Experience" Search Page (http://www.sharedexperience.org/experiencesearch.lasso)*

Address http://www.sharedexperience.org/experiencesearch.lasso Go

Search the Shared Experience Pages

Try searching using different words in the form fields. You can narrow the search by selecting a specific cancer type from the "LIST All" pop-up menu below, then after viewing results, return to this page and try other words in different fields to broaden or narrow your searches.

Search Experiences Database	
Cancer Type:	BREAST
Diagnosis:	DCIS
Chemo Drugs:	Tamoxifen
Treatment:	mastectomy, radiation
Quality of Life:	Fine
Information Gathering:	Susan Love, Internet
General Comments:	Never give up hope
Page Number:	

Find All - or type keywords above and click: Search Reset

As can be seen in Figure 3, to search the website's database of patients' stories of their illness, or, alternatively, to add one's personal story to the existing database, one has to choose a particular cancer type from a dropdown list. Rather than using an open form, one enters one's personal story into a structured form, which contains a range of possible "stories": Acute Myeloid Leukemia, Brain Tumors, Breast Cancer and so forth. Below this drop-down list there are open text fields for categories such as "diagnosis," "chemo drugs," "treatment," "quality of life" and so forth, to allow entry of particular details. Visually, these categories appear as text boxes. They are static "grids" of meanings that help the patient—both as storyteller and as reader—to impose meaningful order on the incoherent experience of her illness. This technical structure, which is repeated in different variations in different websites,[18] helps to turn the flux of the experience into narrative and provides the patient with a tool to master events that are ordinarily beyond her control. Each patient's personal story can be read as an independent text that configures different events in a temporal order and directs them toward a conclusion.

This personal stories database can also be seen as a tool for information seeking. A search of the database can translate the stories into forms of information. As well as displaying each personal story as an independent textual unit, the database can also fragment personal stories into small units of information that are clustered under a fixed range of generic topics such as "diagnosis," "treatment" or "quality of life." The poster dismantles her experience into "chunks" of information that she can fit and insert into the table's rows. In other words, rather than reading a posting vertically, as a story with a beginning, a middle and an end, the reader can view many postings in parallel, reading information on one aspect, for instance "treatment," horizontally across many postings. In this way, the process of storytelling can actually be transformed into a process of information seeking.

Another online element that provides patients with a sequential and spatial framework to organize their experience is the actual interaction with fellow sufferers through message boards and e-mail correspondence. The process of locating one's experience in time and space is based primarily on the interaction between "veteran" online participants (who are also veteran in the experience of illness and treatments) and "newcomer" patients. Women who join the discussion on message boards and similar breast cancer online forums are often welcomed by "veterans." The work of "welcoming" entails the implicit provision of a sequential framework, to guide the newcomer about the way in which she has to organize her experience. As B relates:

> AOL had some boards for breast cancer. That one had all these people that were there who had been through it or were still going through it and I remember typing in questions there and those people answered me. Somebody answered me right away and then I got hooked on to go and talk to these people. I remember the whole time I was going through the treatment, they would tell me: you've got to do this, and I would tell them tomorrow I'm going to have this, and they would tell me what it was. (B, interview 2)

A posting of a newcomer's story is usually followed by replies from other members—whether on the public space of the message board or privately via e-mail. "Veteran" members draw on their own experience to help the newcomer order her experience. They tell the newcomer what to expect at which stage. For instance, should she get a wig before or after her hair falls out because of the treatments? An issue such as the timing of getting a wig is key to a patient's ability to configure her experience into some kind of framework that she can practically think about and plan actions around.

While B's quote undoubtedly describes information exchange, it consists of more than that. The communicative process that she describes involves an ongoing interaction with her fellow sufferers, which enables her to configure the events she has gone through in the past, is going through in the present, and is about to go through in the future into a comprehensible framework of meaning. Crucially, this framework helped her to order her experience temporally. The temporal dimension is central to the process of storytelling, and it is an element that would be missing if we were to talk about this communication only in terms of information seeking and exchange.

The asynchronous form of the communication is another element that fosters the process of locating patients' experience in time and space. Most of my interviewees have not participated in synchronous forms such as IRCs (Inter Relay Chats). As I explain later, they found them inappropriate for their needs. The poster in an asynchronous interaction addresses the posting she publishes online to certain readers, whom she assumes would not necessarily be present online at the time she posts her message. Consequently, the author unconsciously fills in gaps and orders her account coherently, so that the readers are able to relate to it without the author being necessarily present at the time they read it. What the author has to tell is inevitably made more explicit and coherent, primarily by ordering her experience in time and space, than if it were communicated in a synchronous interaction such as conversation. In other words, the asynchronous context of the communication seems to gear the messages being posted into a narrated form, or at least into a discursive form that is more ordered, coherent and explicit than what would have been posted in a synchronous setting. This does not suggest that all postings on asynchronous forums are narratives, but certainly there is an implicit pressure in asynchronous communicative contexts to produce texts that have narrative components, in particular, a temporal ordering of events.

A useful example of this point is given in the fictional account *Dear Stranger, Dearest Friend* (Katz Becker, 2000). Based on factual research of women with breast cancer and their Internet experiences, the book tells the story of an e-mail friendship that emerges between two breast cancer patients: Susan, a survivor, and Lara, a newly diagnosed patient. They meet on a breast cancer-related message board and develop an intimate exchange of emotions and experiences that gradually extends beyond the mere experience of the illness. Immediately after coming back from a mammogram, where the doctor suspected Lara had breast cancer, Lara e-mails Susan, her veteran fellow sufferer, recounting her experience of the mammogram. She opens her e-mail message by saying:

> I'm tempted to simply skip the details, but I know you'll write with questions about why and how and when, so I'm going to force myself to slow down, *breathe* and tell you what happened, in the order that it happened. (Katz Becker, 2000, p. 87)

The fact that she addresses her text to a certain reader, and the knowledge that her reader would read her message in her absence, "force" the author, as Lara puts it, to order her experience in a coherent sequential framework, that is, to narrate. Indeed, in her e-mail she produces an extremely coherent account that configures the different details of her mammogram experience into a plausible narrative.

"Gluing" of elements by an overriding topic. The procedure of locating one's experience in time and space involves the assignment of importance or significance to the different elements of the account. Their significance derives from their relation to an overriding subject that organizes the story. As White (1980) observes:

> The capacity to envision a set of events as belonging to the same order of meaning requires a metaphysical principle by which to translate difference into similarity. In other words, it requires a "subject" common to all of the *referents* of the various sentences that register events as having occurred. (p. 15, italics in original)

In other words, for a text to become a narrative there has to be an organizing principle of meaning that "glues" the different elements into a whole. The way online communication is thematically structured provides this "glue." The online space is compounded by topics: website names, discussion group names, subject of messages on message boards, e-mail subject headers, and so forth. Every discursive element belongs to a subject, which works as an organizing principle of meaning, allowing patients to envision a set of personal events belonging to the same order of meaning. By so doing, it furnishes them with tools to create a story: to assemble separate elements into a meaningful whole.

In A's experience, for instance, age constituted the overriding principle of meaning. Because she was diagnosed with breast cancer at the age of 31, age constituted the primary factor that governed her experience. She therefore sought a communicative framework that centered on the subject of breast cancer at early age:

> I didn't go to the support group nearby my house, because they were all from different ages,... whereas [at] Young Survivors Coalition [a breast cancer website] they're younger and that was much more comforting, because I was able to interact with people who were at the same age who understood the ... (A, interview 1)

A typed the key words "breast cancer" and "young" into online search engines. This combination constitutes the organizing theme of her experience. It led her to online spaces that would potentially provide her with a relevant framework of meaning, to which she could relate and into which she could fit her experience. Significantly, A highlights the capacity to reach specific forums that are relevant to her personally as highly advantageous, in contrast to the face-to-face support group that was available to her in her geographical area. While a face-to-face support group is, of course, also organized by an overriding theme, it is often too general and hence limited in its capacity to help a patient to make sense of her particular circumstances. In this respect, the embodied nature of a face-to-face support group is constrained, insofar as it depends on the physical location of the patients, rather than on the thematic specificity of their experience.

This significance of the flexibility of the online communication and patients' capacity to find a personalized context of communication is a notion that recurs in patients' accounts, as the following patient stresses in her e-mail account, by using capital letters to signify shouting:

> There is a ton of info on the web—there are also many quacks out there—just like in life, you have to decide what is real, what's valid and what has value FOR YOU PERSONALLY. (E-mail 2)

Even F, who denies the centrality of online participation in the experience of her illness, actually implies in her interview the usefulness and significance of the personalized aspect of the online communication, that is, the capacity to "tailor" the communication "out there" to her personal concerns and needs:

> I guess I'm not that into the Internet thing, except for what I want it for, for specific things. What **I** look for, for specific things (emphasizes 'I'). (F, interview 6)

K's experience (interview 11) seems especially enlightening in this regard. K actually found the dominant online frameworks incompatible with her personal experience. She identified two main frameworks of meaning that govern the online communication of breast cancer; however, she could not relate her experience to either of them:

> I think there is a kind of *terrorizing* of women that's going on around breast cancer on the one hand. And on the other hand, there is an awful *sentimentality* about it. I just felt I couldn't relate to either of those really (laughs). (K, interview 11 [italics added])

Following the failure of "fitting in" to either the terrorizing message or the sentimental one, she quits breast cancer-related online spaces:

> The reason I stopped looking at that stuff and didn't find it useful was that I found that around the time I was interested in having surgery, for instance, it struck me that most of the time what women seem to want to discuss was reconstructive surgery, and particularly on the American sites that seemed to be the norm. There seemed to be no debate about it, it did come across like that.... At the same day [of] the appointment I found out that I've had breast cancer, the consultant actually wanted to start a conversation with me about reconstruction, and I didn't want to have this conversation at all! (K, interview 11)

What K's online experience reveals is patients' capacity not only to choose the frameworks and meanings that are relevant to their experience, but also to eschew those that they find irrelevant and futile. This capacity is seen by many patients as unique, particularly in contrast to offline contexts. In K's experience, in the interaction with the consultant, the latter inflicted upon her the message of reconstructive surgery, which she did not want to hear at that point. Online she could simply avoid messages about this issue. The flexibility of the online communication works both ways: whether to enable a patient to relate her experience to a specific topic or to allow her to avoid altogether the available frameworks of meaning.

The thematic organization of online sites and the capacity for conducting a personalized search prove highly significant in allowing patients a structure for constructing and telling their experience. Of course, these organizing principles are not specifically connected to storytelling. They can equally act as facilitators of other communicative processes. For example, patients often emphasize the advantage of the personalized aspect of online communication in relation to information search rather than to that of storytelling. So it is important to bear in mind that my aim in accounting for these elements is not to claim that they are exclusive to the process of storytelling, but rather to highlight their potential relevance and usefulness in enabling this process, among other communicative scenarios.

Asynchronous environment as a framework for storytelling. In the previous section I focused on the content of the communication. I showed how patients' capacity to personalize the content they encounter online, in order to suit to their personal interests, helps them find a suitable framework for the construction of their story. I now explore the form of communication as a significant factor that directs participants to narrate their experience. More specifically, I argue that the asynchronous character of many of the online settings in which breast cancer patients engage provides them with an accessible framework for the production of their stories.

Women's core engagement in the online communication of breast cancer seems to be in asynchronous, rather than synchronous, environments. While the latter exist, mainly in the form of IRCs,[19] they seem to attract a limited "hard core" of members of online breast cancer groups. Unlike these participants, most women whom I interviewed regard chats as an inappropriate platform for the kind of communication they seek. My interviewees often depicted chats as an "unknown territory" from which they deliberately exclude themselves. Tellingly, when interviewees mentioned chats they often expressed embarrassment. For instance:

> I have never been into one of these chat-room things. I don't plan on going into it. I mean, I've heard some really wild stories! (laughs) I don't see that that would be interesting to me at all. (F, interview 6)

Many women's perception of chats is based on mediated representations of chats such as the discussion on sexual harassment and pedophilia on online chats, rather than an actual personal experience. Their suspicious view of chats seems to channel them to engage in communicating their experience mainly on asynchronous spaces. Even women such as the one quoted below, who are highly computer literate and have actually participated in chats, expressed their reluctance to use chats in relation to their illness:

> I don't go on chat sites because I do not fully understand what is going on in those rooms. I go in to some chat rooms to see what they are talking about but it mostly seems to be people who are angry and need to vent or young people being ignorant. (E-mail 14)

Women look for a place where they can make sense of their experience. The work of making sense requires the patient to "slow down and breathe," as Lara, whom I quoted earlier, writes in her e-mail to Susan (see Katz Becker, 2000, p. 87). Women often stressed the significance of being able to "slow down and breathe" and communicate online at their convenience in terms of time and space:

> I could surf on my own time ... when I was in the right frame of mind ... and when the house was quiet so I could concentrate. (E-mail 7)

> Never had to leave the house & go to the library had it all at my fingertips!!!!! (E-mail 8)

> [T]he benefit of finding that information and support in the comfort of one's own home. (E-mail 24)

> It was comforting to know that I could look up whatever I wanted and do it in my PJs [pajamas] at 3 AM if I felt like it. (E-mail 2)

Chats do not allow one to "slow down and breathe"; they demand instantaneousness and swiftness. In contrast to the nature of synchronous forms of online communication, the "chattiness of e-mail," as one of my interviewees observed (G, interview 7), makes it a "natural vehicle" for women to communicate their experiences. Asynchronous forms, e-mail in particular, constitute an ideal platform for storytelling. On the one hand, they contain a dialogic dimension, which plays a crucial role in motivating women to narrate their experience (an issue that will be developed in the next chapter). The patient orients her writing to a specific other. At the same time, unlike synchronous online conversation, asynchronous settings provide the storyteller with a monologic communicative structure that allows her a relatively high degree of freedom and control. The following extract captures this hybrid nature of asynchronous interaction, as a communicative space that is both monologic and dialogic (the split into two parts is mine, to highlight the idea of duality):

Monologic { When your in this situation you're on such a roller coaster it's nice to calmly sit down and search with out some one over your shoulder. And you don't have to talk to any one at that time. Grieve is a big part of the process and sometimes you just don't know how it will play in it. So there is no pressure.... And you can deal with it on your own time and own way.

Dialogic { But if you need to talk your a click away. (E-mail 25)

Asynchronous forms are spaces where a patient is neither dependent on immediate interaction with others, nor limited in time, or in space, and where she can arrange her thoughts independently and in isolation, before a correspondence starts:

> Probably the best part of the internet is that you need to type your question or feeling before you can share it and sometimes just writing it down is a therapy of its own. (E-mail 21)

In conversation, on the contrary, patients are far more dependent on the reactions of the other participants. The monologic aspect of communication, where the patient does not receive feedback, has been stressed in the literature as a significant component that facilitates the process of storytelling. Writing without a required immediate feedback allows patients to explore their feelings and convey them as a story, in a way that is not always possible in conversation (Carlick and Biley, 2004, p. 312).

In short, the combination of a space that allows participants to "slow down and breathe," that contains both dialogic and monologic qualities, and that is anonymous and disembodied serves as a suitable place for the production of self-narratives. Another key element that facilitates the process of storytelling online is the establishment of the authority of a storyteller.

Establishing the authority of a storyteller

> I am sorry you had to join the ranks of women fighting the dragon. (A message posted by a veteran breast cancer patient-participant on a breast cancer message board, in response to a message of a "newcomer" patient, who has been recently diagnosed)

Images of that kind are not rare on the online pages of breast cancer patients. As discussed in Chapter 3, images of a battle against monsters and dragons are part of the wider dominant cancer narrative (see also Stacey, 1997). The act of narrating and storytelling online, I suggest, enables participants to establish themselves as forceful heroines "fighting the dragon." This process is achieved through the establishment of the patient as a storyteller authority or, to put it differently, as the protagonist who propels the plot of her own illness. The significance of this process lies in the hermeneutic relationship between storytelling and agency (as discussed in Chapter 2): through the act of telling, the authority of the narrative becomes the authority of reality itself. Through the construction of a story, the patient asserts herself as an active agent, informed and involved in the course of her illness and healing. The next quote captures this idea neatly:

> There are women on the message board in all stages of breast cancer. The ones who stick around are the fighters ... those that come on and are passive and feel it's just too hard to fight it, give up and give in to their disease and don't stick around. (E-mail 15)

The author equates patients' active online participation with their active approach to their illness, and vice versa: those who choose the "passive" route and give up their online participation are equally surrendering to the illness. A patient's identity and engagement online, especially in storytelling, are mutually implicated.

For a patient to constitute herself as an active online participant, and thus an active patient, she has to make her participation visible. "Leave your footprints," as the "Shared Experience" website encourages its visitors.[20] Online, writing is the central means to "leave footprints." Of course writing can be involved in various ways of online participation and self-presentation in which patients establish themselves as authorities through text. Storytelling is one such way. Thus the discussion of storytelling should be qualified and understood within the wider context of patients' engagement in various online textual activities in which they seek, whether consciously or not, to assert their agency.

Personal home pages are probably the clearest manifestation of an online space where a breast cancer patient constructs herself as an active agent who propels the story of her illness. One of the informants of this study launched her personal home page, where she traces the experience of her illness and healing. Clearly, her website can be seen as a project of establishing herself as an authority. The slogan she made up is reflective of her attitude: "Only in silence can breast cancer continue to kill." Telling the personal story is seen as the way to cure. The act of voicing one's experience through storytelling promises an illusion: control and mastery of the uncontrollable. Thus, authorship, if you wish, implies authority.

The following extracts from a patient's personal website put a gloss on this argument:

> Welcome to my journey.
> ... Many times I have been asked by authors and journalists just "... what spurred you on?" **I did it for, and by myself**. I wanted the cancer OUT of my body! [emphasis in original].
> ... The amazing aspect of this experience with cancer is that I personally witnessed the power of the universe!

However, individuals' engagement in the establishment of their selves as storyteller authorities goes beyond the explicit manifestation of personal home pages. Arguably, the very individualized and particularized nature of the online experience enhances an "I mode" in which one positions oneself in the center of the story. Consequently, the storyteller often marginalizes or excludes altogether other factors that might constitute driving forces of the plot.

It would be inaccurate to say that women do not give credit to their doctors, their family members and other caregivers in their stories. However, I suggest that the individualized self-centered experience of a woman using the Internet on her own translates, to a certain extent, to her capacity to establish herself as an active heroine fighting the cancer, almost in a Proppian sense. In the interviews I conducted, it is noticeable that women who have not used the Internet personally (those whose husbands or other family members have used it on their behalf) tended to construct themselves in far less active terms than women who have been directly engaged in the experience of storytelling online (on message boards, e-mail or personal home pages). While the latter clearly located themselves at the center, propelling the plot of the course of their illness, the former's accounts often foregrounded their doctors as the central agent of the plot.

Similarly, when asked to reflect on the place of the Internet in the experience of their illness, interviewees often depicted their online experience as insignificant. They marginalized the role the Internet played in coping with the illness: "I'm not that into the Internet thing" (interview 6), "it didn't fulfill my needs" (interview 10), or "there is not much to tell" (e-mail 1). Such comments, however, are often contradicted by what emerges from their accounts as a rich experience of online participation that played a central role in the management of the disease.[21] This could be explained as patients' unconscious attempts to construct themselves as the key exclusive agents who "made it," reducing the role of other possible factors such as the Internet that might have helped them in their battle against cancer.

In this context, the apparent variety of the available voices on the online space and the capacity of one to choose among them paves the way for patients to establish themselves in their own terms, as active agents. As the following patient reflects:

> Originally I went to a support group for women with cancer but found out early that it wasn't for me. Most of the women sat around crying about their situations, yet took no active part in their treatments and just believed whatever their doctor told them.... These were not ignorant women, but I think most of us have been trained to believe that doctors know best. This is the reason I went on the internet to look for a sight where women talked about their experience.... I think I am hoping to find someone who did the same thing as I and had a successful outcome. (E-mail 14)

Even if a patient is satisfied with the medical treatment she gets and pleased with her doctors (which appeared to be the case for most of my interviewees), the online context furnishes a discursive space where patients, implicitly, have more freedom and more opportunities to bring themselves to the fore and establish themselves as self-responsible agents, rather than as passive patients who are dependent on their medical authorities. An example of this observation is provided by L (interview 12). L recounts how, when she used to meet her doctor, she would be often at a loss for words, despite the many questions she had prepared at home. Once she went online, she would look for answers to her questions, whether from other fellow sufferers or from online medical sources of information. In the online space it is easier to take the active role, be it through storytelling or other communicative practices such as information seeking, as in the example of L.

Here, my discussion moves on to the ways in which online communication enables patients to construct closure. As I stress throughout this book, the construction of closure is one of the key aspects of the process of storytelling. The struggle to achieve closure distinguishes storytelling from other communicative processes in which patients engage online, for example, information exchange. While the latter is based on the communication of contained units of information, which by and large have to stand independently and be understandable in themselves, storytelling involves the configuration of separate events into a plausible whole, and their direction towards an ending. The project of a breast cancer patient directing her story towards closure is part of the wider story of survival and cure that governs the discourse of breast cancer (see Chapter 3).

Directing Towards Closure: A Story of Survival

> I am cured but I'm not sure anyone can actually say they are cured when they've had cancer. I AM a survivor, tho. (E-mail 18)

The above perceptive comment shows an awareness of the paradoxical experience of a breast cancer patient. On the one hand, the reality of the illness does not allow final closure, as there is always the risk of recurrence. Since an absolute cure from breast cancer is never guaranteed, one can never completely end the story of one's cancer. At the same time, a patient is constantly seeking to reach an end of the illness, that is, to impose a closure on the story of her cancer.

As encapsulated by the patient cited above, for many patients the way out of this paradox is the adoption of the role of a survivor. The discourse of survival—which is highly central to the culture of breast cancer, as discussed in Chapter 3—does not deny the experience of the illness. Rather, it acknowledges the traumatic experience of the illness and its continuous consequences for one's life in the present. At the same time, however, it insists on a closure of this chapter, stressing the end of the "battle" and the patient's triumph over the cancer. The emphasis is on the future, hope and optimism. The following message of a breast cancer patient captures this duality neatly:

> If my CAT scan next week comes back normal, like expected, my Cancer Treatment Experience is supposed to be finished on April 1st.... Seriously, that's the date of my last radiation treatment! After that, I will be somewhat sunburned and sore cancer survivor!!!!! (Posted on a breast cancer message board)

The above message is an attempt at constructing a closure: the patient announces her arrival at the finish line of her "Cancer Treatment Experience." She thus claims the role of a survivor. At the same time, being a survivor does not imply forgetting the experience of illness. Her sunburned and sore body, and hence her story, are a living testimony of her pain. What is more, while the message is clearly cheerful, hopeful and optimistic towards the future, it is framed as an uncertain situation, using the conditional "if."

The production of a narrative on online sites is one way of enabling a patient to actualize this dialectical role of a survivor. It offers a path out of the pain and, at the same time, a guarantee that it will not be forgotten. In other words, I suggest, the process of storytelling is restorative in that it guarantees the remembering of the experience, and thus remembering as healing, but also writing to forget, or at least contain the experience, by placing it firmly in the past (Stacey, 1997, p. 242). Stacey's (1997) conclusive chapter of her book *Teratologies* unfolds these dialectics very sensitively:

> Do I hesitate to finish this book for fear of what might follow? Has it protected me from death? As long as I keep writing I might indulge in a fantasy of control, of authorship of the narrative trajectory of my health, a fantasy that contradicts my knowledge of my own mortality. Or does this piece of writing display a lingering fear of death's imminence: having said my bit, must I prepare to die?... Or is the writing itself a sign of life: I must still be alive, I am producing—'I write therefore I am'? " (p. 242)

Drawing on Stacey's reflection, I next discuss patients' engagement in writing, and particularly storytelling online. I argue that storytelling online offers patients the possibility to constitute themselves as survivors and perform what Stacey calls a "symptom of not dying."

A Space for Testimony

Patients' online forums constitute spaces for testimony. They provide patients with tools and legitimacy to tell their experience and constitute themselves as "survivors." Take B, for example, who explicitly identifies herself as a breast cancer survivor. In her account of her online participation, she stresses how her survivor identity is constructed upon the commemoration and the celebration of the triumph over cancer, through talking online:

> A couple of people will say: why do you want to talk about that? There are some people, and not even just breast cancer [patients], but relatives and stuff, would say: why don't you just ... it's over and done. Put it behind you. Pretend it never existed. I can never answer that to anybody's satisfaction. It did happen, so you can't just sweep it under the rug and say: no, it never did. (B, interview 2)

A "Queendom" of Survivors

The online interaction on breast cancer websites resembles tribal power relations, where the old and experienced people have a privileged voice.

Breast cancer patients' online spaces are implicitly structured by a hierarchy of voices, where survivors determine the tone. This is not to say that newly diagnosed patients or patients who are in the course of their illness cannot voice their experience. On the contrary, they are encouraged to do so. However, their experiences are not voiced in an open neutral space, but rather one that is dominated and framed by certain key actors, namely survivors, and by a discourse of survival. Indeed, many websites and online communicative forums are effectively run and owned by survivors.

Been there, done that. Underpinning the dominance of survival and the foregrounding of survivors in the discussions on breast cancer online forums is the "been there, done that" principle:

> Tons of information you get from other women who have dealt with BC is different from what the doctor tells you. He tells you what the treatment should do, lists the possible sideeffects, recommends medications to combat the side effects, etc. The ladies have BEEN THERE, DONE THAT—they give you an honest accounting of how it happens, what it feels like, what side effects are and how to handle them. (E-mail 2)

In their interviews, women often stressed the significance of the "been there, done that" component of the representations they encountered online. These representations are first-hand experiential stories produced by their fellow sufferers who went through their illness and won the battle over cancer. They are stories of survival. They emphasize a sense of ending. J's description of her encounter with fellow sufferers' stories on breast cancer online forums illuminates this observation:

> [I]t's comforting to read: oh yes, this is supposed to be happening ... another woman goes through this, you do get a certain matter of strength, because you read things from women, I'm one year out, I'm five years out, I'm eight years out. *You know that there is an end* and these women live healthy normal lives, *it's all over.* (J, interview 10 [italics added])

The stories of women who have "been there" provide patients who go through the illness in the present with the temporal perspective that they lack. They order the different events involved in the experience of illness and configure them toward a closure. As the above quote illustrates, in so doing they help patients who struggle with cancer in the present to configure their own experience in some temporal order. It helps them hold to the idea, however intangible it may seem at that moment, that their own story of illness will also come to a similar happy end. The act of temporal ordering and the imposition of closure, as I discussed in Chapter 2, stands at the heart of storytelling.

The shaping of patients' stories by survivors. It is not only that new patients are influenced by survivors' stories that they read in constructing their own experience; survivors are also actively shaping patients' accounts through their online interaction with breast cancer patients who are going through the course of illness and treatments. This interaction, I suggest, constitutes a situation of "joint authorship" of survivors and patients, who together produce stories online.

The interaction and exchange of experience between fellow sufferers, commonly on message boards or via e-mail, usually occurs between patients going through the illness and survivors who have "been there." The patient who is new to the board initiates the interaction by presenting her experience of diagnosis and illness. This initial account is, of course, not free of influence of the discourses and cultures in which it is embedded. It often contains elements of the dominant meanings of breast cancer that were discussed in Chapter 3, namely, self-help and self-responsibility, hope, survival and agency. However, what it often lacks is a sense of closure. It is an account of a patient in a liminal stage, for whom the future is completely unknown. These postings are often replete with ellipsis points ("..."), question marks and explicit expressions of fears and anxieties. For instance:

> I was hoping you would be able to help me ... when I should get a wig ... should I get it now or wait until later. I have been reading some of the messages and they made me cry ... so many people going through the same thing, how ignorant I was before this and still feel I'm in the dark. I think sometimes I choose to be an ostrich! :) ... My mind is rambling on with things I want to say, a part of me just wants to scream. (A message posted by a breast cancer patient on a message board)

Such postings are a call for experienced patients, who are usually "veteran" participants, to "intervene": to help the inexperienced patient-storyteller to shape her story, and particularly to help her construct a closure, rather than remain an "ostrich," as the above quote puts it. Indeed, the story cited above generated a dozen other patients' stories in response. A (interview 1) conveyed this very well when she proudly told me that the message she posted following her medication treatments engendered nineteen responses. This was the goal of her posting: to prompt the production of other postings that will reassure her she is not alone and help her direct her story towards a desired end.

Survivors' responses guide the patient in terms of practical issues, such as when to get a wig, whether to participate in a clinical trial and how to deal with the kids, but also direct her as to her self-identity and what she should expect of herself. For example:

> Your attitude sounds great. Do not feel bad if some days is not so great. You will have both days where you will be strong and then of course there will be days where you will look elsewhere for strength. (A message posted on a breast cancer message board)

It is fascinating to trace threads of discussion that are composed of an initial posting of a patient who is going through a stage of pain and uncertainty, followed by a chain of stories she gets in response that help her shape her own story, and then view the patient's reformulated story, which carries the "footprints" of the survivors' replies. In fact, the message that was quoted earlier, of a patient who describes herself quite cheerfully as a soon-to-be "sunburned and sore cancer survivor," is a "product" of a joint authorship. The message was first posted on the message board, and then was reshaped by the help of other survivors. As I have been arguing throughout this chapter, this directing and redirecting of patients' accounts toward closure are the essence of the process of storytelling.

The organization of online spaces by themes, structures and symbols of survival. The eminence of the discourse of survival is manifest also in the actual visual and textual ways in which many breast cancer websites are designed. "Young Survivors Coalition," which is a website focusing on breast cancer at an early age, is a good case in point. First and foremost, its name and URL contains the word "survivors." Second, its home page displays a list of words, in different font sizes, namely: "challenge," "inform," "act," "support," "question," "empower," "inspire." These words are all verbs rather than nouns. Typical of the discourse of the "enterprising self" (Rose, 1992), they call on patients to fulfill their potential as agents. They resemble an organizational discourse, as if what comes next were about a business project rather than a personal health project of the self. More particularly, I suggest, this discourse calls on patients to move from "passive" online participation (lurking and reading) to active participation by expressing themselves online and sharing their experience. Using this kind of rhetoric implicitly directs patients to express themselves in similar terms to the ones the website employs, that is, to depict themselves in active terms as "empowered," "active" and "informed." Indeed, many of the patients' postings on that site seem to follow a similar rhetoric and a clearly utopian and inspiring sense of agency.

Another interesting example of how breast cancer websites are structured to direct patients to construct a story of survival can be found on the "Shared Experience" website, which provides its visitors with an electronic form in order to fill in their personal information. While the first pivotal moment in a breast cancer patient's experience is commonly the discovery of a lump in her breast(s), this moment is skipped in the story-form provided on "Shared Experience." The first category to which the participant is asked to refer is "diagnosis." In this way, this structure directs the patient to begin with a moment of certainty. The diagnosis may be a threatening or a frightening moment, yet it is a moment of relative control, compared to the moment of discovery, which is characterized by total uncertainty, lack of information, confusion and anxiety. This decision to skip the discovery and start from diagnosis was made unconsciously by E, the designer of "Shared Experience." However, when asked to reflect on his decision, E actually reveals that the discourse of survival and hope unconsciously underlay his decision:

> Gosh ... should I actually change that? [i.e., add a category of 'discovery' before the one of 'diagnosis'] ... But that would be very scary, wouldn't it? (Interview 5)

In her study of an online discussion group called the Breast Cancer List, Sharf (1997) testifies to the notion that patients' communication seems to be tempered by hope, and "to make this colloquy about living with breast cancer, rather than dying from it" (p. 73).

The ongoing nature of online communication as a sign of survival. As I have stressed thus far, patients' online communication is orientated towards the production of stories of survival. This is a dialectical process: on the one hand, it aims at imposing closure while on the other hand it aims at maintaining a sense of openness and continuity. A key feature that acts to facilitate these dialectics is the ongoing nature of the online communication. Here I depart from accounts such as McLellan's (1997) and Hardey's (2002) that underscore this feature only in view of how it facilitates the emergence of a dynamic, open, unfinished and unruly text. I argue that this aspect is only one side of the coin and that we need to understand the ongoing nature of online communication as a dialectical framework: one that sustains openness, continuity and perhaps unruliness, while at the same time constitutes a structure for the construction of closure(s).

The ongoing nature of online communication furnishes patients with the capacity to constantly rework their story; they can update it, edit it and change it over time. This technical capacity allows them to claim their role as survivors, that is, to effectively confirm and reconfirm: I'm still alive. In fact, women often explicitly use this notion in their online posting as well as in their e-mails. For example, one of the women whom I contacted following a message she originally posted a year before replied in an e-mail that starts with this sentence:

> I am still alive and well in Northern California. (E-mail 15)

The capacity for immediacy of publication, of avoiding the usual lapse of time between experience and book publication, yields a distinct meaning to the act of writing online. A patient can effectively come back to the online space and make herself visible, confirming and reconfirming (both to her readers and to herself): "I write, therefore I am." Indeed, women often revisit online forums to tell their continuing story. By being present online, they claim their survivorship, a year, five years, ten years and even fifteen years after being cured.

The five-year milestone has a particular significance in the context of breast cancer as it is considered to be the threshold of a reduced likelihood of recurrence. Patients often come back to online spaces five years after their diagnosis, even if they have not remained active online all these years, to announce and celebrate the closure of their story: their triumph over cancer. For example, here is an e-mail message I received from one of my interviewees, which she sent to a list of her acquaintances and fellow sufferers:

> Subject: Ready for a smile???
>
> Today is 5 years that I have been cancer free! Woooooo Hoooooooo!!!
>
> I can feel you smiling from here!

Another temporal milestone in which patients often engage in online storytelling is the eve of their annual mammography. The latter is part of the regular follow-up of women who suffered from breast cancer. Commonly, women who retired from online participation once they were "cured" go back online before their mammography "because you get nervous around those times" (B, interview 2). The online space is always there: one can join in, leave and come back at any time. This unlimited availability enables patients to engage in the dialectical process of survival: to open, close and then reopen and reclose their story in their own terms and their own time.

B describes patients' maintenance of their online participation, and particularly online storytelling, even long after they have been cured, as a "knock-on-wood" effect:

> I think that a lot of the people that have survived it.... I think ... they're proud of it, part of it is like a 'knock-on-wood'. If I say I had it 20 years ago, and I keep coming [to the online support group] maybe I won't ever get that. (Interview 2)

Perhaps, as B observes, patients unconsciously regard the sustenance of an ongoing online participation, and of storytelling in particular, as an "insurance" policy. This policy enables them to manage the difficult task of bringing an end to an experience that in fact cannot be ever fully closed, as there is always the risk of recurrence. The emphasis on patients' experience of the illness as never fixed and determined but, rather, a "work-in-progress" (Love, 2000, p. xvii; see Chapter 3), seems to be facilitated and endorsed by their capacity to engage in the online space on an ongoing basis—in particular, their capacity to construct and reconstruct their self-narrative: to change, edit, and update, on an immediate basis, at any time.

Writing as the Triumph Over the Body

> The joy of writing.
> The power of preserving.
> Revenge of a mortal hand.
>
> *The Joy of Writing*/Wislawa Szymborska (1993)

Szymborska's poem eloquently implies how the act of writing entails a triumph of the text over the body: the actual writing has the power of making the mortal immortal. The notion of the act of writing as an attempt to subjugate the body to the text emerges as a central theme in breast cancer patients' accounts of their writing and storytelling on the Internet.

The idea of writing as a way to enable the body to prevail appears extremely interesting in the context of the online space, given the latter's profoundly disembodied character. To put it simply, a patient seeks to contain (if not subjugate) her bodily experience by presenting herself in writing, in a disembodied medium. At first sight, bridging this tension between an embodied experience and a disembodied space might seem impossible. However, attending closely to the voices of the individuals engaged in this experience, we realize that it is precisely the production of an embodied account on a disembodied discursive space that enables them to take the "revenge of their mortal hand," as the following account illustrates. In it, a breast cancer patient recounts how, during the surgery she went through, she was planning the way she would describe her experience in writing, in her online breast cancer diary:

> The anticipation to write makes me happy and keeps me occupied. Yesterday I went through transplant surgery, as the surgery takes place, under local anesthetic, on the verge of falling asleep, I went over in my head the way I'll put in writing the event I'm going through, I planned how I will write it, and in what order I'll describe the events. I do it often. (Letter 3)

This story exemplifies how the act of storytelling, especially the ordering of events in time and space—already in its very early stages when the ideas are "cooking" in the author's mind—enables the patient to "leave" her body and disconnect from her corporeal experience. This capacity for displacement and dissociation, through the act of storytelling, has a central role in the patient's therapeutic process. "The analysand is to be witness to his/her own mind" (Schafer, 1980, p. 38). The storyteller can empower herself "by stepping back from the mesmerizing power of events" (Sennett, 1999, p. 12). In other words, by dissociating herself, the patient is able to reflect on her painful situation. Frank (1995) encapsulates this inextricable link between storytelling and dissociation in describing his experience of writing his illness: "I felt written from the outside, but my own voice was doing the writing" (p. 71).

The online environment constitutes an ideal site for this process of dissociation through the act of storytelling. To a large extent, the situation of being behind the screen when one is not physically visible, and where one can remain anonymous, constitutes an appropriate context for one to step back from one's personal experience. As A reflects, for her, remaining anonymous on online forums by using pseudonyms signifies detachment from the cancer:

> Sometimes I'll say Anne or Marie, but ... I find that a lot of young people do want to leave the breast cancer behind. (Interview 1)

Notions of "anonymity" and "disembodiment" in cyberspace are often related to the idea that virtual and fluid identities can exist with no necessary link to the physical body. However, for A, as for many other breast cancer patients, rather than experiencing a "virtual" fluid identity in the postmodern sense, telling her personal intimate story online and at the same time remaining anonymous is a way to "leave the cancer behind" and dissociate herself. This is unlike other contexts of her life in which she is often labeled as the "one with breast cancer" (as she puts it).

In the story *Dear Stranger, Dearest Friend* (Katz Becker, 2000) Lara, a breast cancer patient, writes in her e-mail to her fellow sufferer Susan:

> I still have that *out-of-body* experience from time to time. You know, like I'm watching this happen to me instead of it really happening to me. (Katz Becker, 2000, p. 111, [italics added])

Participants often refer to the postings they published online as if they were an independent entity that exists outside of their bodies and their selves, "floating" in cyberspace. Patients often provide links to other online sites where they published other messages. For instance, a woman who has her personal website sent me an e-mail in which she constantly refers to other online links of her story:

> [S]ee IMPORTANT UPDATES on my website/Updates (E-mail 6)

Another woman, responding to my request for her participation in my study wrote:

> Thank you for your interest, please send me the link to shared experience board, I need to review what I had submitted. (E-mail 29)

In this way, it seems to me, breast cancer patients enact and reenact this out-of-body experience, watching their own story as if it were happening to someone else. The ability to disembody themselves plays a central role in patients' ability to claim themselves as survivors who remember and preserve their painful corporeal experience while being able to leave cancer behind, avenging their mortal hand. I will develop the issue of disembodiment in the following chapters.

The Stop of Storytelling Online as a Sign of Survival

To fully grasp the meanings of the process of patients' storytelling on the online space, it is useful to examine situations in which patients choose to stop their online participation. In particular, I mean to focus on patients' decision to withdraw from writing on online spaces. Why do patients stop engaging in the interpretative work of storytelling?

As I have discussed so far, the act of writing online constitutes a way for patients to claim their identity as survivors: "I write, therefore I am." Interestingly, however, for some patients, at different stages of illness and treatment, stopping their online writing is also a way of conveying their survivorship. A's comment about breast cancer survivors who keep participating in online discussion forums illustrates this observation:

> They're five years survivors and they're still on the Internet?!! (Interview 1)

Earlier in her interview she criticizes more generally breast cancer survivors who remain active in communicating breast cancer, even years after being cured. She implies that retiring from online communication is a sign of survival:

> [T]hat's the problem I think I have with breast cancer survivors. There's something of a victimness about it, you know ... for the rest of their lives, they have this label they wear the pink. (A, interview 1)

What A suggests is that to sustain active online participation, especially through writing and storytelling, is like continuing to wear the pink ribbon, instead of moving on and "leaving cancer behind." For her, once a patient is cured, the motto should be: I don't write, therefore I am." A's perspective is emblematic of the view of many breast cancer patients. For instance:

> [T]he more you talk to people about it the more depressed you would get (F, interview 6)

> When I first got diagnosed, all I did was talked about cancer and researched cancer. Now, I'm in remission, thanks god, I don't want to talk about that at all. I'm so happy to be alive, that I want to live life! I don't want to talk about it. (E, the founder of a cancer website quotes a friend who suffered from breast cancer, interview 5)

Another example is B, who, following her diagnosis, used to post messages on breast cancer message boards, asking other participants about aspects of the illness and its treatment. After she was cured, she stopped participating in discussion on those boards, though she did keep engaging in other kinds of online activities. By disengaging from message boards, and especially from telling her story, B conveys a significant message to herself and to her environment, namely: I am a "patient" no longer. A, too, signed off once she got cured and got back to normal healthy life. She describes the time when she stopped her online participation (in relation to breast cancer) as a moment of a "return to normality":

> I followed that (breast cancer message boards) I'd say for a year and a half, and after that point my menstruation came back, my hair grew in, chemo was over, radiation was over, so I really had no more questions. (A, interview 1)

To some extent, the act of storytelling online as an attempt to regain mundanity had translated into life and had become reality, so she retired from storytelling activities online.

On the other side of the coin is a second reason why patients stop engaging in online forums, particularly by withdrawing from storytelling. Patients often retreat from participating in online forums when they feel that they are incapable of sustaining a "cheerful" story. As discussed in Chapter 3, the motifs of hope and "triumphalism of survivorhood" (Ehrenreich, 2001, p. 1a) are deeply ingrained in the discourse of breast cancer, and women's online stories are governed by these motifs. When a breast cancer patient is incapable of "fitting" her story into this framework, she stops storytelling online. Her decision to stop storytelling is often linked to the actual physical circumstances that technically disable her going online. Many women said that during periods when they were weak from chemotherapy, they usually did not go online or did so only as lurkers rather than as active participants.

In short, patients' decision to disengage from online participation sheds light on the complex meanings of storytelling online. When the perpetuation of the act of storytelling signifies "victimness," as A describes it, stopping this act represents survivorhood—I don't write, therefore I am. When the act of writing represents a sign of life—I write, therefore I am—a patient stops storytelling if she is incapable of claiming herself as truly "alive." Each scenario highlights the centrality of the act of writing in patients' actualization of themselves in the dialectical process of agency and survival.

Conclusions: From Annals to Narratives

> Narrative becomes a *problem* only when we wish to give to *real* events the *form* of story. It is because real events do not offer themselves as stories that their narrativization is so difficult. (White, 1980, p. 4, italics in original)

Patients' experience of breast cancer does not offer itself as a story. Rather, the initial representation of the illness, as it is given by the medical authority, is often closer to the form of "annals": a set of laconic medical details that seem to posses no central subject, no clear relations and no identifiable narrative voice (based on White, 1980). As I showed in the beginning of the chapter, patients represent the moment of diagnosis in a very fragmented and laconic way. In going online and sharing their experience, breast cancer patients often endeavor unconsciously to construct a coherent story that will order their experience in time and place, assign significance to the different elements of their illness by linking them with an organizing principle of meanings and direct them towards closure.

White (1980) views narration and narrativity as the instruments by which the conflicting claims of the imaginary and the real are mediated, arbitrated or resolved in discourse. If we take this view, patients' storytelling online can be seen as a means to bridge the imaginary and the real: it arises out of patients' desire to impose coherence, integrity, order and closure on an experience of life that is rather chaotic, is incoherent and does not allow a final closure. As I have discussed throughout this chapter, this activity is closely entwined with the notion of survival: a dialectical effort to remember and forget, to keep the painful experience open and accessible, while at the same time close it and move on. As I have argued in this chapter, the online environment constitutes a suitable site for patients to mediate and resolve the dialectics of their situation, through, among other processes, the production of stories.

CHAPTER 5

Exchange and Reciprocity

First what you do when you get diagnosed, you look for people who have been through or going through what you do. Then when you're done with it, people contact you. (A, Interview 1)

As the above excerpt of a breast cancer patient's account implies so neatly, a promise of exchange between participants underlies the interaction between patients in the online space. As I discussed in Chapter 2, patients' engagement in exchange online has been framed in various ways. A common agenda has been patients' exchange of information. In particular, studies looked at how patients exchange medical information and first-hand knowledge through different online structures and applications (e.g., Eastin, 2001; McLellan, 1997; Pew Internet & American Life, 2003). Another focus has been patients' exchange of experience and feelings (e.g., Preece and Ghozati, 2001; Sharf, 1997). Drawing upon these frameworks, this chapter develops the discussion on patients' exchange on the Internet by focusing on the activity of storytelling. The intention of this chapter is to enlighten storytelling as central to, embedded in, and enabled by structures and processes of exchange online. Without ignoring other possible frameworks, I show how patients' dynamics of exchange on the Internet enable them to engage in a meaningful process of storytelling, one that endows them with powers to cope with their new situation in life.

The introduction presents how deeply the principle of exchange is embedded in the experience of breast cancer patients' online communication. Following is a characterization of the main features of breast cancer patients' exchange online. I then analyze three key processes that constitute patients' exchange online: (1) engagement and disengagement; (2) anonymity, disembodiment and re-embodiment; and (3) communitas. Each of these processes, I suggest, shapes in significant ways the experience of patients' storytelling. Finally, I close the discussion by highlighting the contribution of the model of storytelling, in comparison to other available models, to our understanding of participants' exchange on the Internet.

Exchange and the Online Communication of Breast Cancer Patients

An examination of breast cancer websites reveals how they are structured to provide a framework of exchange, particularly through storytelling. While these websites encouraged visitors to produce their personal stories, they stress the dialogic, rather than monologic, purpose of the stories:

> Your words are for others who follow after you and the more you describe your experience, the easier it will be for others to relate.[23]

Indeed, patients' online participation exists in a situation of exchange from its early stages. In posting their message online, patients seem to have a kind of a tacit knowledge that there is an audience out there, to read and respond to their posting:

> **I knew** that if I went online, somebody out there would know. (G, interview 7, my emphasis)

> At first, it was comforting to hear other people, you know, you're asking people, especially on BCANs like [a breast cancer bulletin board], something that you noticed, whether it'd be a rash, or waking, nausea.... **You know** that after medication people would respond and that was very comforting. (A, Interview 1, my emphasis)

To follow Blau, who predicated his theory of social exchange on economic motives (Ekeh, 1974, p. 170), underlying patients' engagement in this exchange is their expectation to derive something from this association, to profit and be rewarded in certain ways for their act. While women would rarely articulate their behavior explicitly in terms of profit, most of them did express implicitly the expectation of getting feedback from other patients as their underlying motivation for sharing their experience online. Posting any kind of text on an online site probably entails an expectation of some feedback. However, I suggest, constructing a personal story and communicating it online involves a heavier investment (emotionally, temporally, textually) than say, posting an informative question. Hence the expectation for a reciprocal act, that is, for someone to respond to the posting, is arguably amplified if the message posted is a personal story, rather than other discursive forms such as a short note or a question. This assumption is endorsed by Barthes' (1974) stress of the contractual notion of storytelling. A patient's decision to narrate her experience and tell her story online,

Barthes would have argued, is underpinned by the implicit assumption that she would get "something" in return from her listener(s): a response, a comment, or another story.

Patients often express their expectation for feedback overtly in their postings. Take, for instance, the following excerpt from a posting of a patient on a message board. After telling her readers about her positive diagnosis with breast cancer, the author closes her message with a humorous call for responses:

> Thanks for your continuing words of support. You are the most sensational group of women. Now, enough of this seriousness. Get over on the off-topic[24] and respond to my subject post over there if you there! LOL! [Laughing Out Loud]. (Posted on a breast cancer message board)

Accordingly, when patients receive feedback to their posting, they feel a sense of achievement:

> I got 19 responses so that was very good! [proud] ... People from Australia! Yah! That was good, very good! (A, interview 1)

> I posted that and then I heard from ... a lot of other people e-mailed me after that. People from all over, I mean there was somebody from Canada, you know just from all over! Oregon. (F, interview 6)

> It's [B's online column on breast cancer] averaging like 2,000 hits a month, which I think is fine for just a little column on breast cancer. (B, interview 2)

Yielding a large number of replies, especially from respondents across the globe, constitutes a confirmation that the patient's message has been received, in the technical sense. But more significantly, it is an affirmation that her message came across, and that readers were able to infer its meaning.

Women are often surprised, especially in their first encounters, by the prominence of exchange on breast cancer online spaces:

> I expected to find and did find answers to all my questions from statistics to definitions of doctor's terms that I didn't understand. Something I didn't expect to find were so many people who had been through breast cancer who were so eager to share their experience and be there to encourage others. (E-mail 13)

> I expected to find a lot on the web, what I did find and was not expecting was a HUGE group of breast cancer patients and survivors who became permanent friends. (E-mail 2)

However, very quickly they come to learn about this exchange-based space, and seem to regard it as taken for granted:

> I read the letters from people. I just went by breast cancer, or something like that and then I just read all these different women's letters and then I somehow got into submitting my own letter. (F, interview 6)

What is curious about the way in which women like F describe their decision to engage online is this almost mindless mode that "just" "somehow" got them into submitting their message. After all, people do not disclose an intimate experience such as breast cancer so easily, in a public space, in front of readers whom they do not know. Evidently, in their accounts, women told me how they were reluctant on different occasions to engage in exchange relations, whether in specific online spaces such as chat rooms or offline (e.g., at the workplace). Sharing one's personal story of breast cancer is not a trivial act, hence the significance of exploring why women are motivated to exchange their stories in specific online spaces. For a patient to "somehow get into" disclosing her intimate experience in a public online discursive space (albeit in an anonymous and disembodied fashion), she has to feel comfortable enough and she has to trust the way the exchange works. In particular, she has to trust that her readers would be able to infer the meaning of her story, that they would respond to her posting, and that the "system" would be capable of facilitating this exchange.

How Does Patients' Exchange Online Work?

What follows is a brief characterization of the features of patients' exchange on the Internet. The distinction between the different features is merely analytical and the order of their presentation is arbitrary. These elements exist and take place simultaneously and it is their confluence that creates a framework for patients' interactions. The presentation of these features is the backdrop for getting to grips with the environment in which participants interact, and how it shapes, facilitates and is shaped by their online activities, particularly storytelling.

The exchange occurs mainly between patients. While other actors such as friends, caregivers, family members and medical professionals are also involved in those exchanges, the most prominent actors, quantitatively as well as qualitatively, are patients. Although most websites allow people who are not breast cancer patients to participate in their interactive forums, their spaces are nonetheless implicitly designed almost exclusively for patients. For example, the following are the instructions for participants who want to participate in the 'BCANS' (Breast Cancer Action Nova Scotia) message board:

> Please keep in mind that people posting to the Breast Cancer Action Nova Scotia web site come from all walks of life and from all over the globe and offer a variety of different viewpoints and opinions. *Posters may be be* [sic] *in any stage of breast cancer—newly diagnosed, advanced breast cancer and long time survivors.*[25] (BCANS Board Etiquette & Policy, italics in original)

Ostensibly, the board is open to people "from all walks of life and from all over the globe"; however, effectively it does not allow room for non-patient participants. In this sense, online spaces such as the BCANS website provide a fundamentally different setting of interaction from those of other exchanges in which patients engage. They furnish a basis for an egalitarian communicative space, intended for patients only. This is a significant factor, especially given the prominence of patients' interactions with health professionals, in which power relations are clearly hierarchical. Later in this chapter, I review the claim about the egalitarian dimension of patients' online exchange.

The exchange is transacted through text. Patients' online experience is usually the only textual exchange in which they engage; the rest of their exchanges are oral. The stories patients post online may include non-narrative elements, such as informative questions, or other pieces of information, such as the details of their diagnosis. What distinguishes a story, however, from other kinds of postings is that it constitutes a text that organizes the author's experience in time and space and assembles the different elements of the reported experience into a whole, usually directing them towards an ending or conclusion.

The exchange is voluntary. Online forums would normally have a certain policy and etiquette that instruct participants regarding their participation in the interactive forums. However, these instructions are very general. Overall, the exchange is open insofar as formal obligations or commitment are concerned. There are no formal contractual obligations between the online participants. The obligations incurred in the interaction between patients are not specified, or at least are defined very loosely.

The exchange commonly takes place in asynchronous settings. Such settings include message boards, mailing lists, e-mails, discussion groups and newsgroups. While there are synchronous forms of patients' exchange online such as chat rooms (e.g., OncoChat, BCANS chats), the kind of exchange that facilitates storytelling seems to be fundamentally asynchronous rather than synchronous. Consequently, the time of the exchange is not contained or defined. A patient can contact other patients at any time of the day, and there is no specific time in which a reply to her posting is guaranteed. The time period of the exchange relations is not specified either. Some exchanges are short term, consisting of a few turns only, while others develop into long-term relationships that often last for years.

The exchange takes place on both dyadic and multiparty levels. Exchange between patients often evolves on a multiparty level, usually when a patient posts her message on a public forum such as a message board to an unknown audience of readers. It can then emerge into a multiparticipant discussion and/or, often, to a one-on-one exchange, commonly conducted via e-mail.

The exchange is anonymous and disembodied. Unlike other exchanges in which patients interact during the course of their illness and treatment, the online setting is the only space where their interactions are disembodied and anonymous. Although they may extend into embodied relations (some women, for instance, meet their online pals later in a face-to-face interaction), for the most part, exchange relations emerge, develop and are sustained in a disembodied manner. The disembodied nature of the interaction implies the anonymity of the participants. Some participants reveal their real identity, usually as the interaction evolves; arguably, however, a certain degree of anonymity is sustained as long as the interaction is disembodied. Noticeably, veteran online participants who are often breast cancer survivors, and who participate in online interactive forums on a regular basis, tend to reveal their personal details such as their real name and home address. As I will show later, against much of the writing on disembodiment and anonymity online, which focused on participants' capacity to invent personas and disguise their real identity, these features seem to take quite a different meaning in breast cancer patients' online experience.

Exchange and Storytelling Online

The confluence of these features creates an environment for patients to engage in exchange relations with fellow sufferers. In this section, I explore three key processes that characterize patients' exchange interactions in this environment, showing how they are inextricably interlinked with patients' engagement in storytelling.

Engagement and Disengagement

A key aspect that patients appreciate as special and significant in their exchange online is their capacity to experience a hybrid condition in which they interact, concurrently engaging and disengaging. A key facilitator of this condition is the capacity to lurk. Lurking enables the online participant to be there and yet at the same time not be there: to observe the social interaction and its dynamics, while at the same time remain invisible, without having to interact.

A careful analysis of women's accounts reveals the centrality of lurking in their online engagement. Significantly, most women do not engage in exchanging their experience immediately after their first online encounter. Rather, they usually start participating in breast cancer online interactive forums as lurkers, reading other patients' postings while refraining from voicing their own. Some remain lurkers during the whole course of their illness and it is only after they get cured that they start actively engaging in the exchange. Others start exchanging their experience at earlier stages of the illness. The period of the lurking constitutes a fundamental preparation period for their active participation, particularly in storytelling.

Lurking as a preparatory stage for storytelling exchange. In any interaction, while actors have to have a certain level of trust before they start engaging in the exchange, their ability to judge the actors and the interaction is quite limited prior to the actual exchange. Trust develops mainly as the exchange relations evolve (Blau, 1968). In contrast, in their online relations, patients are capable of establishing a relatively high level of trust in the actors and the form of the relations before they actively engage in the actual exchange. Through lurking, participants gain familiarity with, and consequently trust in, the exchange relations, before actually getting involved in any kind of transaction.

In particular, through lurking, participants become familiar with the common modes of discourse of the interaction. A prominent form of communication they encounter on online forums is storytelling: patients sharing their personal experience in the form of a story. When they start to actively engage in the exchange, they follow the patterns they have learned during their lurking period. This way, they often imitate the way other participants communicate, and produce their own self-narrative. Indeed, personal stories become a taken-for-granted form in patients' online communication. In the interviews I conducted, women often referred to the notion of story as the obvious object of their communication online: "I posted my story," "I read women's stories."

Through reading other participants' stories, patients can get to know and trust their partners in the interaction, without actually having to risk anything. This advantage is particularly notable in relation to face-to-face interactions in which patients engage, such as support groups:

> Originally I went to a support group for women with cancer but found out early that it wasn't for me. Most of the women sat around crying about their situations, yet took no active part in their treatments and just believed whatever their doctors told them.... This is the reason I went on the internet to look for a sight where women talked about their experiences.... Reading these different experiences ... proved very helpful. (E-mail 14)

The capacity to lurk before actually getting involved in exchange relations with other actors enabled this patient to minimize her risks. She could "window-shop" the available communicative spaces, to decide which communicative framework suits her best, without having to actually pay any price. With the face-to-face support group, paying a certain price is inevitable: she had a limited way of knowing the particular nature of that face-to-face support group ("women crying about their situations") without actually engaging in the exchange. Following the lurking period, some patients, like the one cited above, decide to move from passive to active participation, whether by posting a comment, a question, informative text, or a story.

Some participants remain lurkers and decide not to move on to storytelling, or any other active participation that involves posting:

> I didn't ever post any messages.... [I]t just seemed like these women were ... [silence, K thinks] **involved in a form that was about mutual support, it wasn't about having arguments**. (K, interview 11, my emphasis)

K was looking for a critical discussion, informational and rational ("having arguments") rather than engaging in affective discourse like storytelling. However, she could not find it in the online space she visited. Thus, unlike most of the patients I interviewed, for K, lurking was a process of critical reflection on breast cancer online spaces, by which she felt quite alienated. It is precisely the fact that she remained a lurker, and never got into actually exchanging her experience with other patients online, that enabled her to take a critical distance from the interactions that went on in these spaces.

Lurking during exchange. Patients can step back and disengage by lurking also during the actual exchange. Their stepping back does not necessarily result in a ceasing of the relations; they can engage in ongoing exchange relations and yet at the same time, when they choose to, step back from the interaction to the position of a lurker. A few women noted that at certain periods of their illness, particularly when they were physically weak (often during chemotherapy treatments) they did not have the physical and the mental ability to participate actively in online forums. During those periods, patients often find exchange to be a burden.

Yet, at the same time, patients desire a continuity of communication, support and reassurance. Lurking proves invaluable in this respect; it enables patients to keep engaging in the communication, however, as readers rather than as active participants. While they do not produce online messages during these periods, they engage in the reception of others'. The act of reading others' postings, I suggest, is a meaningful part of the wider process in which they engage, of the ongoing construction of their self-narrative. It is part of the self-reflexive and interpretative nature of the process of storytelling; following other stories they encounter, participants weave their understanding of themselves by working and reworking their interpretation of their own biography in the form of a narrative and a story (Giddens, 1991). They may not construct this self-narrative textually, or actually publish it, but through reading others' stories, they negotiate the meanings of their own experience, and reformulate their self-narrative.

So the idea of lurking extends the activity of storytelling also to the reader (listener): the reader too is being transformed, through interpreting her partners' story.[26] This observation is represented in the case of J and K, two breast cancer patients who continued lurking throughout the whole course of their illness and did not post anything online:

> I guess I got the most benefit out of reading women who were five years out, eight years out, ten years out. And were living healthy lives, and had children subsequently, just knowing there was an end to it. (J, interview 10)

> [L]ooking at these sites, I remember just starting to see these other accounts and I'm going through this myself.... One of the things that it really brought home to me, was that I am extremely well-resourced in comparison to lots of women.... Once you start encountering other women's stories, you realize that there are a lot of situations of people actually loosing their incomes, marriages are breaking up, or they are completely on their own, or they're facing a future of never being able to have children or whatever.... I don't know what's going to happen to me.... But I know that I'm well off in comparison with a lot of other women that have had it. (K, interview 11)

Lurking enables patients like J and K to engage in a more latent storytelling, without actually posting a story online and exchanging it with others. By reading others' stories, they reformulate and rework their personal story; they appraise their personal experience and locate it in relation to others. So the act of lurking, particularly reading other patients' postings, feeds into patients' reworking of their personal stories, primarily by validating their personal experience. The following extract demonstrates the significance of lurking for the process of validation and legitimization. A breast cancer patient who returns to her regular online message board after a period of absence writes:

> I didn't use my computer for a few days and was blown away by all the news I missed. Reading this forum has helped by reminding me how normal my feelings are.

In short, even if for different reasons participants are not involved in textually constructing their story and posting it online, it seems that the very act of reading others' stories' online (as lurkers) helps them validate their own situation, and consequently reformulate their self-narrative.

Lurking as a strategy of survival. Finally, many women keep lurking after they get cured. The capacity to be present and at the same time be absent, to concurrently dissociate and associate, fits like hand in glove to the dialectical process of survival. Reading other women's accounts guarantees the lurker the remembering of her own experience (as others' mirror her own), but at the same time it enables her to remain remote from the scene. This "behind the screen" position of lurking, where a patient does not participate in online discussions, is a way for a patient to signify to herself: I am a "patient" no longer. Although patients do not continue actually telling their story in online interactive spaces, their online lurking contributes to the ongoing story they keep telling themselves and their environment, in other sites and contexts of their lives.

More generally, this means that the process of storytelling stretches beyond participants' actual production of a story and its telling in the online space. The act of storytelling can take place in other sites of patients' lives (and not necessarily online); however, the production and construction of their story is shaped, among other factors, by their online experience. For instance, the stories patients tell about themselves in face-to-face support group meetings are often influenced by stories of other patients that they encountered online, often only as lurkers.

Anonymity, Disembodiment and Re-embodiment

> Over time, individual personalities emanate from the BCANS Forum [online message board], without influence of physical form. (Extract from the introduction to the BCANS message board)[27]

Anonymity. Closely interlinked with the experience of lurking and patients' capacity for invisibility is the disembodied and anonymous nature of the online interaction. B's account is a useful starting point for this discussion. Although she personally reveals her real name and identity on the online column that she writes, she acknowledges that anonymity plays a role in encouraging other patients to disclose themselves and participate in her column:

> At least half of the questions at 'Ask me' [her online column], the writer is listed as anonymous.... [M]ost people who are online are very open about whatever they're saying. I don't know if they were that open if they were in person. (B, interview 2)

The author of *Dear Stranger, Dearest Friend* (Katz Becker, 2000), a fictional book on breast cancer patients' e-mail correspondence, supports this observation when she admits that if the characters of her novel, who met as patients on an online forum, had met each other face-to-face, they would have been "more guarded about what they say" (interview with the author). As other studies have shown, anonymity provided by online communication encourages individuals' self-disclosure (Jones, 1998; Rheingold, 1994; Sharf, 1997).

Sennett's observation (2002) regarding the ethnographer's interaction with her unfamiliar informants is particularly illuminating in our context, as it sheds light on the role that anonymity plays in shaping people's stories:

> A speaker is more likely to go into things when talking to a foreigner or stranger than to a familiar. The reason is that the speaker uses the occasion to convert tacit understandings and assumptions into explicit, conscious statements, thereby objectifying and exploring the patterns of behavior for him or herself. (p. 17)

Indeed, as I have already discussed in the previous chapter, the need to write to an anonymous "other" forces the patient to convert her implicit tacit experience into an explicit coherent text. This process was notably evident in the e-mail responses that women sent me upon my request for their participation in my study. My respondents commonly provided a very detailed account, often richer than what I asked for, replete with conscious statements about their illness. Similar statements can be often found on messages posted on breast cancer online boards. The situation of an anonymous exchange gears participants to make sense of their experience in explicit terms, and often drives their account toward some kind of a moral conclusion. In other words, the combination of anonymity and exchange seems to facilitate, if not encourage, participants' engagement in storytelling.

Disembodiment. Crucially, it is not only the anonymous context in which the relations emerge that incites patients to engage in storytelling and disclose their experience in a way they would not have done in a face-to-face situation. The promise of disembodiment also plays a significant role in this situation. The author of *Dear Stranger, Dearest Friend* (Katz Becker, 2000) accounts for this aspect when she describes the nature of the online relationship of the characters of her novel, two breast cancer patients who met online:

> The women talk about how their relationship and how they would have been different. Lara says maybe it's easier to pull your heart out when you know you will never gonna have to run into them at the AMP. And I think that that kind of anonymity is a wonderful thing because it allows you to just say what's on your mind. (Interview with the author of *Dear Stranger, Dearest Friend*)

To fully understand the significance of disembodiment for patients who participate in exchange online, that they "will never gonna have to run into their online pals at the AMP," we need to contextualize it in relation to the wider experience of the illness. Breast cancer is a highly embodied illness. Unlike other types of cancer, which are invisible, breast cancer is located in a clearly demarcated part of the body: the breast. Its discovery is often a result of the patient physically feeling a lump in her breast. The experience of the illness and its treatments is an extremely embodied experience. The self-identity of a breast cancer patient is established to a large extent on the basis of her appearance:

> There's so much cosmetics that occurred: your brows, your eye lashes, your pubic hair, your hair ... I look at the mirror and I wouldn't even recognize myself! (A, interview 1)

The disembodied nature of the online interaction compels the patient to confront the changes she has gone through. Paradoxically, the disembodied setting enforces her to bring in the body by textual means. She has to explicate bodily elements that are tacit in a face-to-face interaction. Spelling out her bodily features (e.g., "I am bald") often leads the patient to a process of self-exploration of her feelings and of behavior. Through spelling out how she looks and what she consequently feels, the patient goes through a process of self-discovery and recognition. Storytelling serves as a particularly useful means in the articulation of this self-reflexive process. For example, through her e-mail correspondence with her online fellow sufferer, and through telling and retelling her experience of going bald, A made sense of her new situation to her online pal and thereby to herself. Given the dramatic changes in her physicality during the illness, her relations with people in her everyday life are fundamentally framed by her appearance:

> It's very difficult, because cosmetically [emphasizes "cosmetically"] that's what people notice. [When] I was first diagnosed I'd wear a wig [whispers] and people would go: something is different!... [B]ut you know, I can't control what other people do or say. (A, interview 1)

Exchanging personal stories online facilitates a different kind of relations. Rather than her physical appearance, the object that embodies a patient's "self" is symbolic, namely, her story. Online, the story is the exclusive conduit of a patient's identity. Unlike embodied situations in her life, where she "cannot control what other people say," because her self-identity is overwhelmed by her appearance, in the disembodied exchange with other online participants, a patient can better control the interaction and what she will receive from her partners in return. A patient's control of the interaction derives from her capacity to control her story. She can choose whether she wants to reveal her identity/story, something many patients describe as very difficult to control in their local community, where the story of their illness spreads though the grapevine. And she can decide what kind of identity she wants to construct, rather than be dependent on her physicality. This capacity provides a patient with a sense of control, especially in comparison to other interactional situations in her life.

That being said, for some patients, the anonymous and disembodied nature of the interaction constitutes a constraint:

> You don't know who these people are, you don't … their opinion or their … evaluation of something.... I don't know who they are. I don't know where they're coming from. So I would sort of need to judge them before I could judge. (J, interview 10)

What J regards as an impediment, that is, the lack of information on her partners of exchange, is often seen by patients as a facilitator. They feel it allows them the freedom to "hit it off" potentially with anybody who was affected by breast cancer, regardless of other identity factors (place of living, class, education):

> Eventually, I think, you just hit it off with some people better than others.... I don't know what it was or why we decided … we have nothing in common. She's this Southern-type Georgia belle person and I'm this rough New Yorker! (B, interview 2)

> I am trusting God to put the "right people" with the "right people." (E-mail 10)

The universal nature of the illness enables breast cancer patients to share their experience with other fellow sufferers beyond cultural, physical, economic and social boundaries. The disembodied nature of the interaction enables patients to overcome constraints that they would have faced in embodied interactions (being judged by their appearance, for instance). At the same time, their self-representation online cannot be and is not naked of their embodied offline identity. Patients' online stories are significantly shaped by offline boundaries. Their online stories are an imprint of their selves, and their selves are a product of various identity factors such as education, geographical location, class, and culture. The author of *Dear Stranger, Dearest Friend* (Katz Becker, 2000) endorses this point when she insists that the characters of her novel, two breast cancer patients who met online and maintain an intensive e-mail correspondence, had to share enough commonalities in order to be able to connect and maintain the exchange-based friendship:

> The only reason that they could become friends is because there were enough similarities that enabled them maintain the e-mail back and forth. If one had been very intelligent and the other one had minimal education, or one was a lesbian who hadn't had the experience of being a parent or being married and that kind of a relationship, then to me, it wouldn't have been realistic, that the other one could really relate to her completely as they did. So in some ways they were similar in that they both were married, they both had responsibilities of children, they both were concerned about their illness is affecting their children, and yet their backgrounds were very different. In my mind their physical appearance was also quite different. I don't think that if they had met or lived in neighboring towns they would have been the kind of women who would have been friends. (Interview with the author of *Dear Stranger, Dearest Friend*)

Patients' preference for a disembodied exchange has another dimension, which is aptly captured by the following excerpt:

> If there was no Internet, I might have chosen to tell the story of cancer and coping through lectures and talks with other patients, however that would have required physical and emotional powers that are not always at my disposal. (Letter 3)

Like the capacity to lurk, at times when a patient is physically and mentally weak, the anonymous and particularly the disembodied nature of exchange online appears highly valuable. The capacity to engage in meaningful exchange relations that do not require physical presence is discussed by many patients as a significant advantage.

Paradoxically as it may sound, it is the lack of involvement and disclosure that is ingrained in the idea of anonymity, that enables the opposite to take place. The fact that one can sit at her home, behind the screen, seemingly with no pressure for commitment and engagement (such that she often has in her local context) encourages her to get involved and committed with greater ease than if it were an embodied interaction. Being able to empathize and reach out for the other, and yet at the same time remain comfortably installed behind the screen, in the comfort of one's home is a key dialectic in patients' online experience. It implies patients' capacity to embrace two opposite feelings at the same time: detachment and empathy, dissociation and camaraderie. G reflects on the emotional detachment that is enabled through patients' disembodied exchange online:

> There's a whole other side to it too, that strangers can give to one another that good friend and family members can't. That's that sort of **emotional detachment**, at least in the beginning.... Once you have your neighbor, your sister, or even somebody who lives in your town, as soon as they start to express their own fears, they're falling apart. You spend so much time trying to comfort them, and that's not what you need! You need somebody who's going to support you, who's going to be strong, and that you're not going to want to look across to see the fear on their face. The Internet gives women the chance to do that. Because even if it's killing [emphasizes 'killing'] you that somebody else is going through a bad time, you can tell them, type them a letter and say: "I'm sitting here, crying for you, that's so bad. I wish there was something I could do to help." (Interview 7, my emphasis)

Re-embodiment. Ironically then, patients enjoy the capacity to distance themselves from their physical presence, while at the same time they try to make themselves present. The act of re-embodiment seems to be especially tied in to the act of storytelling. Storytelling is a highly useful way of making oneself present in the disembodied space. A story provides a discursive framework for the participant to make her body and her self visible. Unlike informational forms where patients post online, a self-narrative is probably the textual form that is most capable of making its author present. What Redford (1986) noticed about the eighteenth-century familiar letter is to a large extent true for the online dialogic narrative: "the voice of the letter-writer makes distance presence" (p. 2). In other words, through the production of online dialogic stories patients pursue a process of re-embodiment: bringing the body into a disembodied space. The following is a typical example from an online narrative in which the storyteller devises different discursive techniques to emphasize the corporal context, and re-embody the disembodied interaction:

> I have never had lymphedema before, so I don't know what to expect. I didn't get one of those sleeves ... last night I started getting a tingle and numbing sensation and it's getting worst today. It doesn't seem swollen, just the "asleep" feeling, like you've slept on your arm. (A posting on a breast cancer message board)

Another common device used in patients' online stories is emoticons, particularly emoticons that signify bodily gestures such as { } to signify hugs, {{{HUGS}}}) to signify intense hugs, or xoxox to signify kisses. There are also common "bodily acronyms" such as "LOL" (Laughing Out Loud), and metonyms like **sniff** (to denote crying). Such emoticons and acronyms can be used in independent messages, not necessarily as part of a narrated account, but they are often incorporated into patients' narratives, endorsing the re-embodiment project that the story pursues as a whole.

This dialectical condition of disembodiment, embodiment and re-embodiment works to enhance a story of survival; it enables patients to talk about their body and other bodies, and thus remember and relive the experience of the illness, while at the same time remain disembodied and detached, as a way of forgetting. In other types of interactions, patients seem to have this capacity to a far lesser extent. Offline, their bodies must be present, especially in their medical encounters in which they cannot escape the body.

Online Communitas

> The camaraderie is amazing, the love and acceptance of each other's differences is almost overwhelming. (E-mail 24)

Perhaps the most central aspect in women's accounts of their online experience is their recognition of a special kind of interrelatedness and bonding that emerges from their exchange with fellow sufferers online. The notion of "communitas" aptly encompasses this experience. Largely borrowing from Buber's concept of community, Turner (1969) introduced the notion of "communitas" to refer to a specific modality of social relationship that emerges recognizably in liminal periods. The liminal phase is one of betwixt and between, neither here nor there, "a moment in and out of time" (p. 96).

Patients often describe themselves as "passengers" who go through a transitional phase: the "journey" of illness. Detached from an earlier fixed point in their social structure, in which they were healthy persons, patients pass through liminality: "a cultural realm that has few or none of the attributes of the past or coming state" (p. 94). The transition entails a move from a set of cultural conditions (health/embodiment/engagement/visibility) to a place where they are "to be fashioned anew and endowed with additional powers to enable them to cope with their new station in life" (p. 95). In this transitional phase "communitas" emerges.

Communitas implies a sense of being "*with* one another of a multitude of persons" (p. 127), with an emphasis on the "spontaneous, immediate, concrete nature of communitas, as opposed to the norm-governed, institutionalised, abstract nature of social structure" (p. 127). Indeed, women often describe their experience of communitas online in relation to, if not in opposition to, institutionalized structures of exchange that they encounter in the context of their illness.

In the remainder of this chapter I discuss how communitas evolves through patients' participation in exchange online, drawing on Turner's anthropological account of "communitas" (1969). I show how patients' liminal condition and their experience of communitas online generate storytelling.[28] This process, as I argue throughout this book, endows them "with additional powers to enable them to cope with their new station in life" (Turner, 1969, p. 95).

Unstructured bonding: Immediacy, spontaneity and quick human interrelatedness. As opposed to institutionalized medical interactions that patients experience in the course of their illness and treatment, the communitas they experience online is largely characterized by spontaneity and immediacy:

> I think you start out when you ask questions and go online to a group, looking for somebody who had, at least the procedure that you're dealing with at that time, whatever it is. When I was having the mastectomy... All I wanted to know is that compartmental of time, did you have a mastectomy, tell me about it. And then when I got the kind of chemo I was having, then I wanted to know that. It didn't have to be the same person. Eventually, I think, you just hit it off with some people better than others. Some people also wanted just to ask their questions, and they would discuss their subjects again. Get your information, and then they want no connection. (B, interview 2)

Beyond the general expectation of reciprocity, the nature of the exchange is unspecified and unstructured: there is not a specified type of actor who is expected to give feedback ("you just hit it off with some people better than others"); there is no obligation to sustain the exchange on a long-term basis ("It didn't have to be the same person"); and there is even no clear obligation for truly mutual exchange, insofar as some participants act instrumentally and cease the exchange once they get what they want. These characteristics are not distinctive to storytelling. In fact, B's account describes these qualities in relation to what might be seen as a countercase to storytelling, namely a brief, straightforward and instrumental information seeking ("get your information and then they want no connection"). Immediacy and spontaneity, I suggest, characterize the nature of patients' online communication in general, and apply to a diversity of communicative processes, from short-term information seeking to elaborate ongoing storytelling.

The immediate character of the online communitas has particular significance for patients' liminal condition. In their encounters with the medical institutions, patients are often made to wait without knowing what is to happen and when (Frankenberg, 1992). Thus, the immediate nature of the online communication, of "being a click away" from other fellow suffers with whom a patient can share her experience without having to wait, plays a key role in patients' coping. The communitas that emerges online represents a sense of being *with* one another, on a spontaneous, immediate and concrete level. Unlike other kinds of communitas patients may experience, in order to experience online communitas patients do not have to be confined to a particular time or space:

> The idea that the women can reach out to each other whatever the day or time.... You can go online when it's convenient, you're not tied to a support group that meets every Monday at 7 o'clock. You're not feeling well, not feeling up to getting dressed, putting clothes on getting into your car, you can still benefit from online support which is always there and **you can do it when you can do it.** (G, interview 7, my emphasis)

This special kind of communitas enables storytelling on a "you can do it when you can do it" basis: a patient can create and publish her story any time, and there is potentially a witness to her story any time. This is unlike the stories patients tell in other areas of their lives, particularly in front of their doctors, where their listeners are available at fixed, planned and nonimmediate times and places. The accounts women tell their doctors are usually well structured and prepared in advance. Women told me how they used to plan in detail what they would tell their doctors during their consultation, taking notes and arranging their thoughts and questions as coherently as possible. Given the fixed and limited time and space they have for their interaction with their doctors, patients produce accounts that aim to cover as much as possible and capture the here and now.

By contrast, the nature of accounts that patients tell online is less "condensed": they usually do not attempt to capture the "whole story," here and now, in its entirety, but rather represent part of the patients' experience, which is often followed by more messages that are continuously produced. The fact that the space for storytelling is constantly available, with potential listeners at any time, allows the stories to be produced across time. The unfolding story is being established on an ongoing basis through the process of exchange with others; an initial short message can be elaborated and formulated into a richer and more coherent self-narrative.

Generalized exchange and communal storytelling. It is through this communicative chain of stories that communitas emerges. The primary mechanism that facilitates the creation of a chain of stories, and thus communitas, is the structural organization of messages posted on electronic boards along threads. An online thread links different messages by organizing them under an umbrella topic. In this way, several different postings, often composed by two or more patients, are aggregated into a "metanarrative." The following thread, taken from a breast cancer message board, exemplifies this idea. Note how a message about the relationship between a patient, her cancer, and her mother (posting 1) develops into a story of another patient about her cancer, her family and the Internet (posting 2), closed (albeit never sealed, as one could always reopen this thread by adding one's story) by a story of a third poster about her cancer and her friendship with her online fellow sufferer (posting 3):[29]

Subject: MOMS SAY THE DARNDEST THINGS ... WITHOUT THINKING

[Posting 1]
Yesterday, just my Mom and I went to ... a ... craft store.... I came across over 100 angels and had tears come to my eyes. I just stood there looking at all of them. My mom said, what's wrong, with you? and Why are you crying in this store? I told her, that everytime I see an angel, it reminds me of my ... cancer. She just said, I shouldn't LOOK FOR THEM. I told her, that I love angels, because, even thought, it was a bad time in my life, it was a blessing, too. I think that just about, knocked her off her feet. She said, You are glad you got cancer? I said, no, but I'm glad it happened to meand [me and] not my sister, or her or anyone else in our family. Then, I said, I have so many friends that I love, so much and they all have helped me, in ways they will never know. Then she had to sit down, she was confused.... Well just who are these new people that you say that you love??? I said, it was all of you, who are reading this, now. But, she says, you have never even, met these people and haven't had the time to really know, who they are...Yes, Mom I have. I have them all in a special place in my heart.... It was a very, special day, cause, it was about, my MOM, my CANCER and all my new FRIENDS.... That cancer, made me find, all of you.... hugs & love, Nina.

[Posting 2]
What a sweet message. It's nice when you can spend time with your mom and get along so good. My mom drives me crazy, and my kids

don't even want to be with my mother. I'm so glad that I found these boards to chat on too. I don't know what I'd do without them. My husband was telling me that maybe we should unhook the Internet and I told him noway, nohow. I'm not about to give up my Internet. Well, talk to you later. Jean

[Posting 3]
Wow Nina **sniff** (reaches for tissues). One thing I have found since I have had this "affliction" is missing having my Mother to share it all with. Keep those precious memories, they are important. PLEASE say "hello" to your mother from me here ... seeing I don't have a mother. Show her the calendar too, then she will see what friends you have!!!!! Carol
(*Breast Cancer Online: In Our Own Words*, 2003, pp. 26–27)[30]

While each independent message does not necessarily constitute a story in its own right (for example, posting 3 in the above quote clearly cannot be considered a narrative), the act of exchange and the structure of a thread create, I suggest, a wider story. In this sense, the whole is more than simply the sum of its component parts; from the aggregation of the different messages into a thread, a story emerges: a constellation of different parts into a whole. Such "chains" are based on the implicit principle that once a personal account is introduced into the public space of a breast cancer message online forum, negotiations over its meaning start to take place. Other participants in that space respond to the author's posting, either on the public forum (e.g., by posting messages on a message board), or via e-mail, contacting the poster directly and privately. In so doing, they join in the act of producing a story.

This process resembles an oral situation of "communal storytelling" (Ricoeur, 1980), "collaboratively crafted by many different voices along the way" (McLellan, 1997, p. 98). The idea of storytelling as a communal action implies that, through its recitation, a personal story is incorporated into a communal communication, and it is through the communicative event that emerges that a closure is constructed.

Such communal storytelling is predicated upon what Ekeh (1974) calls "the Law of Extended Credit": a credit mentality where individuals have faith that they will take care of others and will be taken care of in return, although not necessarily by the same people. This kind of "generalized exchange," as Lévi-Strauss (1969) contends, operates on the basis of trust; individuals usually do not receive benefits from those to whom they provided benefit. The following excerpts are testament to the kind of univocal reciprocity between breast cancer patients in online spaces:

> [E]very month I am doctoring somewhere, I end up turning into a basket case. All I have to do is get on there [BCANS online message board] and say I've got an apt. [appointment] coming up and I'm overwhelmed with responses and wishes. These ladies have all been there where I am now, and got through by talking it out with each other. (E-mail 19)

> All of the ladies on the AOL thing [breast cancer message board], most of them, when I go back every once in a while, go to the board, a lot of them have been out for 10, 20 years. This is their commitment to go back and help the new people. (B, interview 2)

> After I was done with chemotherapy I stopped really doing the Internet, but then people were contacting me who were going through, and wanted to find what lies ahead. I still keep in touch with one girl. (A, interview 1)

Egalitarianism and hierarchy

> **One family of women**
> Although we branch out all over the planet, we are a single family sharing unified roots.... [T]his forum is a source of simple sustenance for those whose lives have been touched by breast cancer. Where does a woman turn when her world is torn asunder with the dreaded diagnosis? (*Breast Cancer Online: In Our Own Words*, 2003, p. 7)[31]

The metaphor of a family, which is often used in breast cancer patients' online spaces, implies a strong emphasis on the egalitarian and homogenous dimension of patients' online communication. On the other hand, like in any family, there is a certain hierarchy that underpins the relations between its members. As I argued in Chapter 4, breast cancer online spaces are "queendoms" of survivors, where survivors rule the discursive space and determine its orientation.

The character of the online communication facilitates and enhances the egalitarian dimension of communitas. First, the anonymous disembodied character of patients' online communication furnishes an ideal platform for the exercise of egalitarian relationships. As I have discussed earlier in this chapter, anonymity and disembodiment give participants the capacity to interact while overcoming conventional identity factors that would have otherwise determined power relations in very significant ways. Second, as I noted in the beginning of the chapter, breast cancer online spaces are structured for the participation of patients only. Although occasionally actors such as caregivers and family members do participate in those spaces, the core of the communication belongs almost exclusively to the patients. Third, breast cancer patients' online forums utilize different mechanisms to focus the discussion only on aspects of the illness, avoiding "extracurricular" issues that might undermine the common experience-based communication. The BCANS Forum, for example, directs postings that are not dealing with breast cancer to a secondary "off-topic" message board. This enables designating certain kinds of discourse to certain communicative spaces, so that consequently uniformity and homogeneity are sustained in subtle but effective ways.

This kind of egalitarian and uniform exchange is significantly different from other kinds of exchange relations in which patients engage in the course of their illness, particularly their exchange with medical professionals. While the latter is predicated upon clear definitions of power, patients' exchange online offers a potentially nonhierarchical structure of relations. Indeed, women often compare and contrast their exchange online relations with online fellow sufferers to their face-to-face exchanges with nonpatient actors, particularly with their doctors. They highlight the significance of the common experience as a basis for genuine communitas:

> It has been my experience that only those who have had an intimate relationship with cancer can truly understand the stages a newly diagnosed patient will go through. (E-mail 24)

However, the nonhierarchical dimension of patients' communitas online is only one side of the coin. The communitas between patients is fundamentally based on a clear hierarchical order, by which online newcomers who are newly diagnosed patients follow their instructors, online veterans who are breast cancer survivors. The interactions in breast cancer online spaces seem to follow the principle that Turner (1969) described in relation to rites of passage and the emergence of communitas: "The high could not be high unless the low existed, and he who is high must experience what it is like to be low" (p. 97). As the following patient alludes:

> Within the OncoChat and the breast cancer listserv Internet groups, the responses to my questions and expressions of fear and angst have been met with understanding. There is always someone who has walked in my shoes already and can say, with honesty and compassion, "I know just how you feel." (E-mail 24)

To be able to "walk in one's shoes," with honesty and compassion, there has to be a certain order of relations: on top of the hierarchy are those who have "been there done that," that is, veteran patients, commonly occupying the title of "survivors." Their role is to mentor newcomers who are relatively new in their "breast cancer journey." The latter are in the liminal stage; they must experience what it is like to be low, in order to be high, that is, to emerge and reach their mentors' position. This hierarchical principle frames, in significant ways, the communitas that is developed among patients online.

Online mentoring is a voluntary pattern of survivors who remain online—even years after being cured—to welcome newly diagnosed women, and to guide them through the course of their illness. The implicit working assumption is that, one day, when those newly diagnosed become survivors, they will do the same. It is primarily on the basis of this "extended credit" framework of mentoring that a considerable sense of contract between the fellow sufferers emerges:

> So, my friend Nicole, she had mastectomy and hysterectomy … she is ahead of me in the reconstruction, she has the reconstruction done, and so she gives me feedback. It's kind of like a "pecking order," because her, and me and then my friend Nancy… (A, Interview 1)

Having said that, the idea of a "pecking order" of mentoring between patients is not unique to the online communication. Indeed, many of my interviewees had a mentor during their illness, outside of the online space, and later, when they got cured, they often mentored newly diagnosed patients. The distinctiveness of the online context lies in the way mentoring is enacted: in a disembodied fashion, through the medium of writing. Take, for instance, the way Susan, in the fictional book *Dear Stranger, Dearest Friend* (Katz Becker, 2000), acts as a mentor to Lara, a newly diagnosed patient, through e-mail correspondence:

> Dear Lara,
>
> {{{ }}} Those are hugs. Cute, huh? Stick with me kid, I'll teach you all kinds of neat Netspeak. (p. 26)

Susan is capable of acting as an online mentor, mothering Lara the "kid," not only because she (Susan) is a breast cancer survivor, but crucially because she is also a veteran active online participant. As Lara goes through the course of her illness and treatments, Susan teaches her not only about breast cancer but also about the discursive rules of communicating breast cancer online. These rules consist not just of medical jargon and terminology, but also of specific forms and styles of expressions, such as the emoticon of {{{HUGS}}}. These are discursive devices that are characteristic of the culture of breast cancer online. To be able to participate in the exchange in this community, one must have some knowledge of the discourse and the norms that govern it.

One of the things Susan teaches Lara is to communicate her illness through storytelling. I have already shown a couple of examples, in the previous chapter, of how Lara works on the narration of her experience in her e-mails to Susan. As their correspondence progresses, Lara becomes an experienced storyteller of her experience. Hence, Susan's role of mentor is twofold: she is Lara's guide to the breast cancer journey and concomitantly her instructor on the online journey.

Online writing, especially storytelling, has interesting implications for the development and sustainability of the mentor-protégée relationship. The following (fictional) excerpt, in which Susan inserts her comment into a bit from Lara's previous e-mail, demonstrates this point:

> From: Susan_P@aol.com
> To: cre8f1@mindspring.com
>
> On 11-29 cre8f1@mindspring.com wrote:
> > (Please, God, help me to raise Wendy to be a more forceful
> > and confident woman and not a dishrag like her mom. Amen)
>
> Now cut that out. You are not a dishrag. A dishrag would not have immediately called her internist for more information. You took action and are not to be condemned. (Katz Becker, 2000, p. 62)

Susan creatively uses her capacity to edit Lara's textual self-presentation to help her reformulate her self-account and reassure her of her decision to get a second opinion about her diagnosis. Susan is rewriting—both technically and substantively—her fellow sufferer's story. After Lara got the definite news she has cancer, Susan wrote her:

> So now that you think you've heard the worst possible news in the world ("It's cancer"), let me switch into my "I'm a survivor [...]".
>
> - Breast cancer does *not* mean you're going to die. I can't repeat that often enough.
> - Breast cancer is *not* synonymous with mastectomy. (Lumpectomies with radiation have been proved as effective as mastectomies for long-term survival. Example: Me!)
> - Breast cancer does *not* necessarily mean you'll even need chemotherapy. (Katz Becker, 2000, p. 105)

In the latter example, Susan employs simple technical capacities enabled in e-mail writing, such as using bullet points or emphasizing certain words by *italicizing* them, to switch Lara's narrative from one of "cancer" into one of "survival." The form of bullet points visually gives the story a clear order, attributing to the content a sense of validity and formality (a sense a breast cancer patient lacks, in the face of the uncertainty imposed by the news of her diagnosis). These bullet points represent, if you wish, the legitimate building blocks of a breast cancer narrative, that is, of a story of survival. E-mail seems to furnish an ideal platform for a mutual reconstruction of their self-narratives: the veteran patient, through exchange, helps her protégée to reformulate her story into one of survival. In so doing, she reconstitutes and reaffirms herself as a survivor.

Susan and Lara's relation exemplifies the way Brooks (1994, p. 57) characterized a teller-listener relation, as simultaneously one of collaboration and struggle: "collaboration toward the creation of the coherent and explanatory text, yet struggle over its interpretation, and over its very constitution." Asynchronous disembodied textual settings such as e-mail provide a useful space for the sustainability of this collaboration/struggle process. Each actor is on her own, detached spatially and temporally from her online partner, free to construct her personal account, under ideal individualistic conditions ("without someone over your shoulder," as put by one of my interviewees). At the same time, the teller and the listener share the same discursive space; they literally share a single electronic sheet, on which they can struggle over each other's interpretation, by means of editing, referring and commenting.

Communitas evolves through these mutual acts of online storytelling. Yet as both Blau (1968) and Turner (1969) recognize, exchange relations often become institutionalized, and the spontaneity and immediacy of communitas can seldom be maintained for very long. Indeed, there are several examples of how mentoring becomes structured in fairly formal kinds of online schemes. One such example is "Chemo-angel," an online form by which patients are assigned fellow sufferers as online pals with whom they can correspond and exchange experience. There is an online team of breast cancer survivors who runs this service and monitors the assignment of "chemo-angels" to patients. As described in the following online account:

> I also have a chemoangel who was assigned to me for one-to-one support. She e-mails me weekly and we have a nice relationship going. The chemoangel group tries to match you up to an appropriate angel and they got me a good one! (E-mail 11)

Another way in which exchange relationships and communitas between breast cancer patients become institutionalized is when survivors become "semi-experts" who write on their experience. Examples can be found in patients' personal web pages, patients' online journals, and other kinds of online columns that patients write on a regular basis. B describes the online breast cancer column she writes:

> For the column.... Mostly, you can logon and they show you how many hits you have. It's averaging like 2,000 hits a month, which I think is fine for just a little column on breast cancer.... Now, at the beginning, there are obviously faithful readers, because they know when it comes out, it comes out every other Sunday, and there's always like 50 hits, for the new article the next day. But, and it's a wide variety, one is about diagnosis, one is about mastectomy, there's a couple about chemotherapy. Consistently over the year, you go back and the pages that had the most hits are the ones about chemotherapy, the ones about radiation. It's the ones about the things that people are going to have to go through: the treatments.... I did one on celebrities with breast cancer. The ones that people read the most, when they come and find the column, they go either to ones about what they're going to go through ... the treatment (B, interview 2)

B's relationship with her readers, to whom she refers throughout her interview as "the people" or "the general public," becomes more like a producer-consumer relationship than one of equal fellow sufferers. Her authorship infers authority, and it is being reconfirmed through the communal act of storytelling; her readers respond to her semiofficial online story, and she responds in return.

Turner argues that the institutionalization of relations erodes spontaneity and genuine human contact. For him, the institutionalization of relations generates a less "genuine" and "authentic" communitas. However, the evidence from patients' experience does not necessarily conform to this conclusion. Even institutionalized relations, such as those between the author of an online journal and her readers, or between a mentor allocated to a specific protégée online, seem to entail a genuine and spontaneous sense of bonding.

Whether spontaneous or institutionalized, the message conveyed in many breast cancer patients' online spaces that is that there are no shortcuts; one has to go through the complete journey in order to be high, that is, to reach the status of a survivor and get reincorporated into the normal healthy social structure. This "journey" dovetails with the journey of the illness and the journey of online communication. And storytelling constitutes a central means in completing this journey and reaching the moment of re-aggregation (à la van Gennep, 1960).

Conclusions

As we saw in this chapter, breast cancer patients engage in a process of disembodied, anonymous and textual exchange with fellow sufferers. This process generates feelings of bonding, sisterhood, camaraderie, and strong empathy among the participants, inviting patients to locate their personal experience in relation to that of others, and consequently validate and legitimize their personal experience. Storytelling, as I argued in this chapter, is a central element in facilitating this process.

I do not want to suggest that the kinds of interaction presented in this chapter are the only possible types. I have explicitly acknowledged that patients' exchange online involves a variety of communicative processes, and that storytelling is only one of them. Nor do I wish to celebrate the online space as the ultimate communicative space for the materialization of communitas and exchange between patients. As I have shown throughout the chapter, in specific contexts, and for specific individuals, exchange on the Internet might be constraining or irrelevant. However, in separating out the main interactional features involved in patients' exchange online, we are better able to recognize the richness of these processes, and understand their significance and distinctiveness.

If we tried to explain patients' exchange and storytelling online with any of the existing models that were discussed in Chapter 2, we would have found them fairly limited. The information-seeking paradigm would have failed to account for the affective dimension that is so central in patients' interactions, and for modes of discourse that are not purely informational, such as self-narratives, that are at the heart of participants' exchange. For example, the discussion of the issue of trust in the majority of studies of health-related online interactions (e.g., McLellan, 1997) remains restricted to the informational level, chiefly concerned with the aspect of the trustworthiness and credibility of the information that is being transmitted. The analysis presented in this chapter suggests that trust is not restricted to the information being transmitted in patients' exchanges online. Beyond the issue of information and its content, patients also require and acquire trust in the actual human communication and particularly in the processes and structures that facilitate it, such as, for example, storytelling. I have shown how personal stories constitute a communicative form through which trust evolves between patients online and how the particular properties of their exchange online render trustworthy the narratives that patients produce.

The model of self-presentation would have fallen short in capturing the dialogic aspect of the communication, and the particular qualities it takes. As I demonstrated, patients' participation in breast cancer online spaces is more than individuals' engagement in their self-formation and self-presentation. It involves a strong collective dimension, and elicits practices like communal storytelling and social forms like communitas. The conversational paradigm and existing models of online community exchange, on the other hand, would have suffered from the opposite limitation. While stressing the communal and dialogic characteristics of participants' interactions, they would not have been able to account for the significant monologic aspect of participants' exchange. The act of lurking, which I discussed in depth, is a clear example of a monologic, one-way act that nevertheless plays a central role in facilitating and driving exchange between participants.

Furthermore, the analysis of breast cancer patients' exchange and storytelling casts critical light on the presumed inevitable link between exchange and embodiment. As I argued in Chapter 2, the underlying normative agenda of research on CMC has been to large extent the need to restore a body-to-body dialogic relationship. And indeed, notions of presence and embodiment lurk in most of the traditional theories of social exchange. However, in line with more recent studies of CMC (e.g., Baym, 2000; Hine, 2000) the analysis has shown that for breast cancer patients, disembodiment is often facilitating rather than constraining. As we saw, the production of a self-narrative and its telling in a disembodied space can allow patients to avoid constraints that they often face in embodied interactions in their lives, while at the same time enable them to get involved in meaningful interactions, representing themselves textually, by telling a story.

Another important issue that arises from the analysis is that participants' exchange on the Internet can be both inclusive and excluding. On the one hand, as the analysis has shown, participants' engagement in storytelling online is radically public, democratically inclusive and indifferent to all patients, unlike expert medical modes of discourse from which patients are often excluded. The inclusive dimension is particularly augmented by the anonymity of the participants. At the same time, as a few examples have shown, patients' storytelling online can also be selective, working as a mechanism of social exclusion. Patients like K, who want to use a different form of discourse, rather than her personal narrative, and exchange different types of content from those that constitute the mainstream discourses that dominate breast cancer online spaces, often find themselves excluded from the communicative process.

CHAPTER 6

Negotiating Public and Private

One of my face-to-face interviews (with A, a 31-year-old breast cancer patient) took place on "Victory Day," the breast cancer survivors' annual celebration of their victory over cancer, marked by different events across the United States. The train that I took from New York on my way to meet A was called the "Victory train," a regularly scheduled train with specific cabins for breast cancer survivors who are picked up on the way. There are public announcements about Victory Day at every stop. All breast cancer survivors who go on the train wear special T-shirts representing the event. Their cabins are decorated with pink balloons, denoting the pink ribbon. Along the way, local supporters wait on the platforms, welcoming the survivors with signs and posters. A, who gave me directions for the venue of our meeting, knew that the train I would need to take is the "Victory train." In one of the e-mail messages she sent me before our meeting she wrote:

> On Saturday there is a train coming from Penn. station [in NYC] picking up all breast cancer survivors and it is called the Victory train. They have it once a year.... **I don't participate in these things because I am more private**. (My emphasis)

Throughout the interview too, she stressed that she does not participate in this kind of event because she is "more private." For A, such breast cancer-related activities, which are outdoor and embodied, are considered a violation of the boundaries between the private and the public. In contrast, to her, the online space represents a private setting, where she has participated quite actively, sharing the personal story of her illness with disembodied fellow sufferers.

This anecdote from my fieldwork introduces the core concern of this chapter: how patients' online activities, particularly storytelling, enable them to negotiate the meanings of public and private in the experience of their illness, and what consequences this process has for their coping.

In this chapter I show how, through storytelling online, among other processes, patients can redefine orientations of public and private. On the one hand, the act of producing a self-narrative and publishing it online constitutes a clear way of transferring a private experience into a public form. In this sense, storytelling online is a way of moving from private to public. At the same time, storytelling online facilitates new ways for patients to construct their privacy and meanings of the "private" in their lives. It constitutes a way to redefine, and perhaps even reclaim, the private realm of their lives. As such, storytelling online constitutes a potential process for transformation: enabling patients to move from private to public and back. It is through an active crafting of boundaries and definitions of the relations between "private" and "public" in their lives that patients tell themselves and their environment who they are. This is a key process in patients' identity self-formation.

The inquiry of this chapter connects to the broader concern of researchers with exploring the forms in individuals' online participation that enable the negotiation of the private and the public:

> [A] continuum of forms of being and acting together is growing from the technology of the Internet.... The challenge to analysts is to understand and appreciate the significance of these various forms of transcending the narrowly private existence and navigating the social world for individual participants, for society at large and for the shaping of the Internet. (Bakardjieva, 2003, p. 294)

More generally, the discussion of this chapter connects to the wider concern with the relation between the public and the private as a central feature of social life, and the role of the media in individuals' management of this relation. The critical literature on public and private is immense and it is obviously beyond the scope of this chapter. The intention of this chapter is to highlight the private/public relation as it emerges in patients' online experience, particularly in the process of storytelling.

However, before moving on to this task, I want to contextualize the focus of this chapter by briefly discussing the private/public issue in relation to patients' coping with chronic illness, and breast cancer in particular. Modern Western culture portrays illness as a private problem bounded to the individual (Potts, 2000, p. 102). On the other hand, there is a strong unifying factor of illness: medical discourses tend to group all sufferers into a homogenous category defined by the disease (Lorde, 1980). Thus, patients find themselves having to manage the boundaries of private and public in their lives as a central process in their coping with the illness.

This dialectical relation between the private and the public has a particular resonance in the case of breast cancer. As discussed in Chapter 3, the central thread in the history of breast cancer has been the move of the disease from the private realm to the public arena: from a disease sealed off from public discourse and public awareness to being "the biggest disease on the cultural map" (Ehrenreich, 2001, p. 1a). There is a growing tendency towards the "privatization" of breast cancer (Leopold, 1999). This trend is endorsed by the emphasis on self-exams and self-detection, which constructs the disease as a woman's private problem and responsibility. At the same time, as Leopold observes, "There is no public forum now in which breast cancer is not at home" (Leopold, 1999, p. 2). The fight against breast cancer is depicted as a collective endeavor, not only of women but also of society as a whole.[32] As Potts (2000) demonstrates in her account of breast cancer autobiographical narratives, patients' personal narratives encapsulate this "double stranding" of the disease, that is, being simultaneously private and public.

The following discussion explores the manifestations of this double stranding in patients' storytelling online. It presents five dimensions, each representing an aspect of storytelling online through which patients can negotiate the differing meanings of and connections between the public and the private in their lives.[33] These meanings may seem dichotomous, depicting what is "private" as oppositional to what is "public." However, as Warner (2002) notes, meanings of private and public are not simple oppositions. In fact, the contexts of public and private overlap, and "most things are private in one sense and public in another" (p. 30). In exploring each dimension, I demonstrate how the act of making a story and telling it online might facilitate these dialectics.

Redefining Space and Time

Time and space function as a segmenting principle, helping people to segregate the private and the public spheres of their lives from one another. Zerubavel (1981) accentuates the centrality of time (which can be extended to space)34 to the definition and regulation of social involvement, commitment and accessibility:

> Our life is socially organized and temporally [as well as spatially] structured in such a way that, whereas during some time periods we must be accessible to others, there are time periods during which we may be legitimately inaccessible to them. (p. 142; the bracketed text is mine; it is included to extend the scope of our discussion also to space)

So, certain spaces and time periods carry specific meanings of the public and the private, which become taken-for-granted meanings of social life (Warner, 2002; Zerubavel, 1981).

However, the experience of chronic illnesses like breast cancer challenges in significant ways mundane meanings in patients' everyday lives, including commonsensical meanings of private and public in relation to certain spaces and time periods. Consequently, whether consciously or nor, patients are involved in an attempt to redefine these meanings, to reconstruct boundaries of private and public places and times in their lives. The online environment furnishes a central site where this project takes place. In particular, the act of storytelling online appears to be a means for participants to "rewrite" space and time as a way of redefining their lives' boundaries of private and public.

Rewriting Space

In their engagement in storytelling online, participants seem to negotiate two key spaces: the body and the home. Both spaces are associated in patients' quotidian practices with the private. However, in face of the illness, their meanings are likely to be altered. The making of a story and its telling online is a process that can enable them to construct new meanings of these spaces.

The body. To a large extent, the experience of breast cancer expropriates patients' bodies from the private sphere into the public realm. The breast, a bodily site invested with meanings of the private (restricted to the sight of very few, concealed and extremely personal), is transformed through the medical procedure of treatment into a public object. Storytelling online, I suggest, can serve as a means of negotiating the new meanings of the body: reproducing and reconfirming its "publicness", while at the same time struggling to bring it back into the private sphere and, by extension, to bring back one's self from public to private.

One of the clearest ways through which the act of writing online claims the body as public is the use of vivid, textual, corporeal descriptions. Patients post online messages in which they describe their bodies in a very graphical fashion. For example:

> I've now had 4x epirubicin and cyclophosamide (and will now have 4 x taxol)—I found that I lost varying amounts of hair at different stages in the three weeks between treatments—I used the cold cap for the 1st 3 treatments—but not the last one. Pre chemo I decided not to pluck/wax/shave so started with quite thick eyebrows—and still have eyebrows—although I did lose a few each treatment in my 2nd week post chemo. It really hasn't made much of an impact on the brows (but apparently the taxol will), I have noticed that this time (ie 2nd week post treatment 4) I have a few lower lashes missing. (A message posted by a breast cancer patient on a message board)

As in the above example, "writing the body" online can be done in a fairly informative format, often as a report. Other patients choose to communicate their corporeal experience in a narrated form. They do it by linking the different bodily experiences they went through along a temporal (often chronological) framework that leads the description to some closure. Some participants also extend the textual act of "writing the body" into a use of visual materials, by incorporating photographs of their bodies into their online postings (e.g., pictures of mastectomies or reconstructed breasts). In this way, their online stories, among other discursive and visual forms, act as a kind of an extension of their bodies.

This line of argument is, of course, quite familiar in recent writing on CMC. There has been substantive discussion of individuals' self-presentation, especially with regard to personal web pages (Chandler, 1998; Hardey, 2002; Hine, 2001), and more generally about the implications of displaying the body in a disembodied environment (e.g., Campbell, 2003; Millar, 1998; Sundén, 2003; Terry and Calvert, 1997). In the health context, Pitts (2004) recently explored how women with breast cancer negotiate identity and definitions of situation in disembodied space, through reading and writing online. Drawing on these works, I suggest looking at individuals' presentation of their selves and their bodies online as a way of extending their most private space into the public space. More particularly, I suggest complementing these accounts by focusing on storytelling as a key practice in this process, that is, storytelling online as a way of asserting the private body as public.

At the same time, online participation, and particularly publishing one's story online, works in the other direction too: as a means to reclaim the body as private. A's account (interview 1) illustrates this point usefully. In her interview, A related six key sites where she shares, deliberately or otherwise, her experience of breast cancer: (1) outdoor spaces such as the "Victory train," where breast cancer patients advocate the fight against breast cancer by communicating their personal experiences and performing bodily activities (e.g., walks, races); (2) her local community (e.g., local grocery, the street, etc.); (3) her workplace; (4) the diner where we had our interview; (5) online interactive spaces such as the BCANs discussion forum,[35] where she participated quite actively; and (6) her home, where she continuously confronts the reality of her illness, by telling, among other things, the story of her illness to herself, her husband and other intimates with whom she interacts in this space.

Each of the above six spaces could be located somewhere along a hypothetical continuum whose polarities are "private" and "public."[36] Of course, the polarities are never absolute and total: each space contains both private and public elements. Thus, the significance of each space derives from its relational position to the others. So too the meaning of the online space is defined in relation to the other spaces:

Figure 4 *The Meaning of Online Space on a Public–Private Axis*

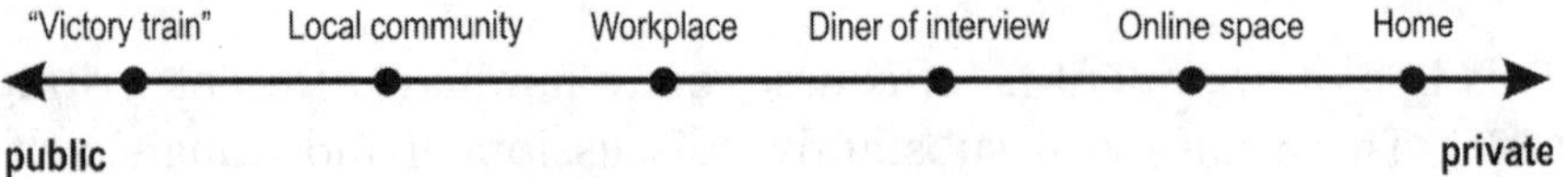

At one extreme are spaces such as the Victory train (public transportation), which signify for A a clear public space. At the other extreme is the space of her home, whose boundaries delineate A's private sphere. Breast cancer is an experience that she regards as totally private. Therefore, for her, it can and should be experienced only in those spaces that are considered private—hence her claim for a clear-cut separation (with which I opened the chapter) between spaces such as the public train and private spaces where she can "display" and experience her illness.

Indeed, after her diagnosis, A wanted to contain her experience within the boundaries of her most private sphere:

> I just really grieved, I didn't really want to read the words "cancer" when I first got diagnosed, I didn't want anyone to say it, just wanted to put my head in the pillow and cry "why me?" (Interview 1)

However, at a later stage A wanted to interact; she wanted to communicate the experience of her illness. Therefore, the private space of the home appeared insufficient; the separation between the illness and the public space could not be sustained. The act of going online and telling her story was an act of "going public": A had to take her head out of the pillow, and necessarily break down the boundaries of her private sphere. On the hypothetical continuum of private and public spaces depicted in Figure 4, this means that she had to move to the left, from the extreme of privacy, that is, her home, to a less private space. At the same time, she kept struggling to preserve her privacy. Hence, she sought a space that would enable her to enjoy both worlds: to tell the story of her body, and thereby make it visible and public, while concurrently remaining with her head in the pillow to protect her privacy and stay out of public touch.

Telling the story of her illness in the online space enables this "middle hybrid." On the one hand, she insists that:

> This [experience of breast cancer] is not information to share, no one should know that. It's a very personal thing. (A, interview 1)

At the same time, she admits sharing her personal experience of breast cancer in several interactive online forums. Significantly, she does not see any contradiction between her perception of breast cancer as an issue that should not be shared publicly and her engagement in storytelling online. She found the online space a site that enabled her to share her experience and, at the same time, remain private. It allowed her to engage in various communicative processes, and produce different discursive modes. She posted information and shared her story; she read others' postings, and published her own. The variety of these communicative opportunities, storytelling being one of them, helps patients like A to manage the public and the private, and to maintain this duality.

The key to explaining A's conception of the online space as a private space is, of course, the aspect of disembodiment. A implicitly highlights the link between disembodiment and privacy when she contrasts her online participation to other breast cancer survivors who "go around wearing breast cancer T-shirts." A regards the latter kind of activity as a highly embodied act that violates the boundaries between public and private. Online participation, on the other hand, she sees as enabling the maintenance of these boundaries. Another patient reflects on the distinctiveness of online communication as a way to transcend, on the one hand, the disembodiment and physical isolation from the public sphere, while at the same time maintain privacy:

> It [the Internet] is a great way [to] avoid becoming isolated—which is so common for cancer patients as either you don't feel well due to surgery or chemo or radiation. or you don't always look good (I am bald now for the duration of the chemo tx) or just you don't feel like being social for whatever reason. The computer is a great alternative to face-to-face encounters with people at a time when you really value your privacy. (E-mail 11)

Of course, disembodiment is a general feature of the online experience rather than one that is specific to the activity of storytelling. However, I suggest that the combination of the capacity for self-disclosure in a form of a story and in a disembodied fashion has particular appeal and value to many participants. I develop this claim in the following discussion of the redefinition of private/public boundaries around the space of the home.

The home. A second key space that is associated in patients' lives with the relation between public and private is the home. During the course of treatment, patients are often physically confined to their home. Consequently, they are unable to unrestrictedly move between the domestic space of the home (private) and the space outside the home (public). As a result, they look for ways to bring the public home: to regain some access to the public, but in a way that would not necessitate embodied access.

In this context, online communication appears very useful, and even crucial for some. The following comment neatly captures the quality of online communication whereby a patient can participate in the public sphere and exercise a public discussion while physically remaining within her private sphere. The split of the sentence into two parts is mine, to demonstrate the duality of public and private:

Public	{ The internet is a place where treatments, definitions, and explanations
Private	{ can be explored in the privacy of one's home. (E-mail 26)

Bakardjieva (2003) describes this practice as "immobile socialization," in contrast to the condition of "mobile privatization" that implies great physical mobility but a home-centered way of living.[37] I argue that the activities of breast cancer patients online, and particularly storytelling, show that actually “immobile socialization” and “mobile privatization” are two sides of the same coin. On the one hand, posting messages online, especially personal narratives, is an attempt at “immobile socialization,” that is, a movement from private to public. Like the woman quoted on page 136 (e-mail 11), patients share their experience on the online space to connect and reach out, beyond the confines of their home. “If you can’t get over the fence then you go ‘under,’” one of the women wrote in her e-mail to me, referring to her online engagement as a way to overcome her physical immobility (e-mail 8). The Internet connection replaces the car; online written communication replaces face-to-face interaction.

At the same time, patients equally reflect on the significance of being able to move in the other direction—that is, from public to private—and to reassert the meanings of the home as a private space:

> It was comforting to know that I could look up whatever I wanted and do it in my PJs [pajamas] at 3 AM if I felt like it. (E-mail 2)

> When your in this situation you’re on such a roller coaster it’s nice to calmly sit down and search.... And you can deal with it on your own time and own way. (E-mail 25)

> The home computer has pretty much replaced the local library as far as doing research and looking for information [is concerned], so it [going online] was the logical thing to do. (E-mail 15)

In this sense, patients’ online communication could be seen as a resolution of “mobile privatization”: offering them mobility at once (sharing their private experiences in a public space), and a home-centered experience, allowing the sustenance of meanings and feelings of confidence, comfort, convenience and privacy.

Rewriting Time

Participants’ negotiations of meanings of private and public in their lives are visible not only in relation to space but also in relation to time. Here, too, the negotiation of the two realms works in both directions, and often concurrently: from private to public, and from public to private.

Private time is deliberately designed to prevent, or at least to discourage, the formation of human contact and to separate people from one another. Public time, on the other hand, is deliberately meant to promote the establishment of human contact and to draw people together (Zerubavel, 1981, p. 143). By going online from home to interact with others, especially at unconventional times, patients unconsciously transform the private time of home into a public time. In their accounts, women often stressed that they tend to go online to share their experience and look for information particularly during late-night hours, times that are commonly associated with the private sphere.

At the same time, however, the very same practice can be a way of reclaiming private time. Through interacting online, some patients seek to reestablish "time preserves" in which they have the right to be inaccessible.[38] Claiming private time "shields" is a particularly meaningful effort for patients, since they "are always socially accessible, and have no time whatsoever within which they can screen out nonintimates" (Zerubavel, 1981, p. 143). Patients seek to reclaim their right to be inaccessible, to re-appropriate the control over their private time. Online communication, and particularly the capacity for lurking (as discussed in the previous chapter), is one way by which patients can exercise this right. G alludes to this idea:

> If someone is giving you the story of her life and you're interested, you can read. And if you're not, you don't have to! You can just skip it and move on to what you want to know. (Interview 7)

Patients' attempts to reclaim their private time are also highly gendered. Women often regarded their online activity as a time devoted solely to themselves, a release from the other times of their everyday lives, where they often act as caregivers concerned with others. Storytelling, among other online activities, often at late hours, delineates for many patients a private space and a private time that are focused on themselves rather than others. Here again, the disembodied and anonymous nature of the communication enables patients to negotiate the public and the private. It allows them the freedom to be inaccessible, without having their behavior considered inappropriate. Unlike other contexts in which patients have "to go through social niceties," as G (interview 7) puts it, online, the definitions of what is an appropriate or inappropriate time for communication are much more blurred. In this context, storytelling online often becomes a more flexible and easy experience than that of storytelling in other contexts of patients' lives, for example, in a face-to-face support group, where a patient must be bodily accessible and so cannot simply tell her story and disappear.

Establishing the Common and the Unique

Another way that storytelling online enables patients to negotiate meanings of private and public relates to the tension between the common and the particular. Through storytelling online, patients can experience the story of their illness as both common and unique. Generally speaking, the public is associated with the common and the general, whereas the private usually represents the particular and the unique. The stories patients produce and tell online help them frame their experience as an endemic one. At the same time, through the very same process, they come to think of their experience as highly special and unique. The following discussion focuses on the ways in which the act of storytelling online facilitates and is embedded in this dialectical process.

The Common Cancer

"The Common Cancer" is the title of a poem written by one of my interviewees.[39] It neatly captures the idea that the story of one's illness shares a lot of commonalities with that of others, and that "It's not that it's so terribly unique," as another interviewee commented:

> There are so many [breast cancer stories] out there! ... Who am I? Why would they be curious to read my story? It's not that it's so terribly unique, but it's also part of why I wanted to tell it. Because it's not so terribly unique! Yes, it's a little unique, maybe the misdiagnosis, but you know what, a lot of women get misdiagnosed! I really felt this could be the everyman, or the everywoman's story. (G, interview 7)

As G reflects, storytelling (whether online or offline) is a way for a patient to frame her personal experience as the "everywoman's story," to come to realize that it is a common experience that other women go through too. This realization happens not only through active telling but also through reading others' stories. For instance, newly diagnosed patients might have been aware of the statistics indicating the high prevalence of the disease among women; however, it is usually only when they literally encountered actual stories of other patients that they could truly experience a sense of commonality. Through reading others' stories, patients seek what Yalom (1970) calls "universality": the realization that others have similar problems. This is true of the stage of diagnosis and also of other moments throughout the illness and treatment experience. For example:

> [W]hen the chemo starts, some physical change goes on your body and it's nice to go on and see that other women have gone through that. (J, interview 10)

The process of storytelling online, enabled by participants' exchange, provides a means to transform a private and unique experience into a public and common discourse. It does so by directing the teller to locate her experience in relation to the other, to locate her own experience within a repertoire of other existing stories. In making this argument I particularly draw on Somers' (1994) discussion of the two key constituents that underpin the positioning of the private in relation to the public in narratives: historicity and relationality. Applied to this study, these concepts imply that through the construction of narratives online a patient can locate herself in relation to other women, on a continuum of experiences, and in relation to the history of the disease. Next, I explore how storytelling online works to facilitate this, and what forms the elements of historicity and relationality take in breast cancer Internet sites.

The structure of the World Wide Web. The first aspect that seems to enable patients to locate their private experience almost inevitably in relation to a public context is the way the online space is structured. The online space is all encompassing: it concentrates a wide range of symbolic materials in a highly accessible way, on an immediate basis. In the process of constructing their message, patients often appropriate different materials that are available in the discursive space, incorporating them into their self-narrative, in a very immediate and direct fashion. For example, when a patient writes an e-mail or posts a message on a message board, she often incorporates elements that she encountered elsewhere on the World Wide Web. In the following example the patient incorporates statistics of breast cancer (public discursive materials) into her e-mail message (private discourse):

> Susan, let's face it, the odds that I am currently hitting are much less than 30%. To recap:
>
> - 80% of the time lumps are benign. (Not mine.)
> - More than half of all breast cancers happen in women over age 60. (Not mine.)
> - Exercise and a low-fat diet are supposed to help reduce a woman's risk. (Not mine.)

- Pregnancy and breast-feeding reduce risk. (Not mine.)
- Beginning menstruation late reduces risk. (Not mine.)
- And doesn't low alcohol consumption also reduce risk? (Not mine.)

Do you see a pattern emerging? And let's not forget, I have no family history of breast cancer although I know that most people (85%) who develop BC don't have family history either. (Katz Becker, 2000, p. 117)

In the example above, the author might have appropriated information from a statistical section of a breast cancer website into the body of the electronic sheet of her message. Technically, patients usually first go through informative (and, less often, commercial) features before getting to the interactive forums where they publish their account. Subsequently, whether consciously or not, they incorporate pieces from the information they encountered online (as well as offline) into the message they post. In this way, a patient's private story relates to the bigger story, the "grand narrative," if you wish, of breast cancer. Patients' online narratives become an integral part of a public discursive framework.

Visually, whether patients' stories are ordered in discussion group threads[40] or in the form of a table,[41] their organization on the screen generates historicity and relationality. Although each message is posted as a singular unique text, graphically it is inevitably "historicized"; it does not stand as a singular, private, unique and independent message, but rather becomes part of a continuum of experiences.

In short, the all-encompassing nature of websites and the visual structure of the World Wide Web, which consist of links to an enormous range of symbolic materials, augment the relationality and historicity of patients' online postings. Private texts of self-disclosures are contextualized in time and space and become part of public discursive space and meanings.

Putting a private experience into a public form. Another way that commonality is enhanced online is by inserting a private experience into a publicly available online form. Patients are often asked to put their personal experience of diagnosis, illness and treatment into a standard electronic form. The idea that a personal disclosure is transmitted into an impersonal public form transforms something that is private and special into something that is public and common. The "Shared Experience" website that was mentioned in previous chapters is perhaps the best example of the ways in which this process occurs. To enter a personal account, the author has to insert her text into an electronic form that is divided into different categories. This structure turns the unique into common, requiring the author to adapt her personal experience to existing categories of similarity. The display of patients' different stories appears in tabular format. The table's columns are the different categories (diagnosis, treatment, quality of life, etc.) and its rows are the personal stories.

Figure 5 *"Shared Experience" Cancer Stories Table (http://www.sharedexperience.org/experiencelist.lasso)*

Page Number	Cancer Type	Diagnosis	Chemo Drugs	Treatment	Quality of Life	Information Gathering	General Comments
4053...	BREAST	In 2001 at age 41, my wife was diagnosed with Duct...	Doing the Dose Dense regimen at the Mayo Clinic in...	Stated above. She had a chest film and blood work ...	Chemo has gone very well. She gets tired easily bu...	My wife did much of the research the first time ar...	We have a very supportive church family who have b...
4040	BREAST	April 16 2002--my first born child's 12 birthday....	fe5u? Epirubison & ? Every 3 weeks for 6 trea...	Lumpectomy April 18,2002--Intensive Chemotherapy ...	I'm Alive—What else is there? Really I have had...	Some of my poetry; Hope it helps in some way ...	It seem's much more recent, but It was perhaps the...
4018	BREAST	Diagnosed on November 7, 2002 with medullary high	Adriamycin and Cytoxan...	Lumpectomy, 4 cycles AC chemo and currently	Fatigue. I had it before the cancer was found and ...	Joined the local cancer support group. This	I think it is very important to have

The table conveys a message of similarity. What organizes the screen are the different categories that unify the different stories. As I discussed in Chapter 4, structuring patients' experiences in this table transforms complete stories, which have a beginning, a middle and an end, into fragmented units of information. This structure of an informative table enables the personal to become public and to enhance its legitimacy and acceptance. It is through the transformation of the personal narrative into general information that the unique becomes common, and that the private becomes legitimate. In this sense, this table can be seen as a collective disclosure: it is not only a collection of private unique experiences but also a kind of general scheme of breast cancer and its different manifestations.

Comparison with others' experiences. The structure of exchange, in which patients' communication is embedded, enhances explicit relations and comparisons between patients' experiences. Authors often refer in their messages to other texts they have read, positioning themselves as similar to, or different from them. It is through the implicit act of comparison between the different stories that the boundaries of the private and the public are negotiated, and that consequently the teller (as much as the listener) gains legitimization and confirmation for her story. Given the vast quantity of patients' stories online, a patient often finds other stories that relate a worse experience than hers. Thus, women often described their encounter with fellow sufferers' online experiences as a meaningful reassurance of their own situation. For example:

> When I went to the Internet it was just strictly for my own knowledge to see how many women had experienced this problem. And it was just shocking, really! You just don't imagine that … a lot of them were worse than I did, I mean I was lucky. (F, interview 6)

Seeing her story integrated into a table, a list or a thread that consists of numerous (often hundreds) of other similar stories, a patient is capable of connecting her private self to the public world. K neatly summarizes this idea when she says:

> [M]aybe that's what you want, you want the kind of distillation, rather than lots of individual experiences. [laughs] … which are all going to be very different, anyway. Perhaps you just want the general information. (K, interview 11)

Disembodiment and anonymity. The disembodied and anonymous environment where patients' storytelling takes place enhances the idea of generality and commonality. It blurs what makes an oral story distinctive: the embodied identity of the teller. Disembodiment has a homogenizing effect insofar as it erases any uniqueness that derives from bodily appearance. Crucially, however, this is not an argument about disembodiment as enabling participants to disconnect from their physical "real" identities. Patients' online stories have both authors and addressees who are connected by a common experience. The common experience, enhanced by the lack of physical contact, marginalizes the significance of differences between the stories and their authors, and emphasizes their commonality. This is not to deny the space for multiple and changing nature of identities within a disembodied textual environment. However, in many breast cancer online spaces there is an emphasis on the creation of a large repertoire of experiences and the similarity between them.

So the diversity of patients' experiences and the differences between them are one side of the coin:

> The camaraderie is amazing, the love and acceptance of each other's differences is almost overwhelming. (E-mail 24)

At the same time, breast cancer patients' Internet sites, and especially the stories published on them, are not just about "each other's difference." In fact, to a large extent the promise of love and acceptance lies in the sameness between patients' experiences. The similar character of the different personal stories enables their authors to communicate, and for camaraderie between them to develop.

While the homogenizing public dimension of breast cancer sites, and storytelling in particular, is enabling for many patients, for others it may be rather constraining. Those patients find it difficult to transform their private experience into a story on a public online space. They also often find it difficult to relate to the sheer quantity of stories and information available on online spaces:

> [T]here's so much out there, and you only want to hear what applies to you. I don't want to hear about stage 3 to stage 4 … I just want to know what's going to happen to *me* [emphasizes "me"], and it's very hard to find that. (J, interview 10)

J, for instance, who is quoted above, did not engage in storytelling online. She went online mainly for information seeking, and even this activity was limited in its extent. Although she is a very verbose storyteller (judging by her interview with me), she preferred sharing the experience of her illness only within what she considered private spaces: at home, with friends, and even at her local synagogue. K, too, found breast cancer online sites inappropriate to communicate her illness experience. However, unlike J, for K the problem was not with the generality of the stories and information, and their overwhelming amount. For K, the main limitation was the opposite: the narrowness of the material she encountered online. She found the existing repertoire of discourses and stories in online spaces extremely limited, and therefore could not meaningfully relate her experience online. In her interview she told me that she was particularly looking for an alternative kind of discourse to that of personal stories. She wanted to engage in a critical, rational and argumentative discussion, and not in an experiential, subjective and personal discourse. However, she could mainly find the latter: personal stories that are about participants' attempts to establish their own "narrative truth" (Spence, 1982; see Chapter 3). These online stories usually did not engage with "objective" medical truth, but rather focused on individuals' subjective experiences. By no means do I suggest that a more critical discourse on medical treatments and options, of the kind K was looking for, does not exist online. Nevertheless, from my observation of patients' sites and the analysis of their accounts, it seems to me that the availability and significance of this kind of discourse are still quite limited.[42]

The Unique Cancer

The other side of the coin is that women regard the stories they tell online as extremely personal, special and thus private. As Potts (2000) argues more generally about breast cancer autobiographical narratives: "while the texts tell a *shared* story, breaking down the isolation of women's experiences of breast cancer with an assertion of the connective and collective, they also assert the unique and *individualized* self" (p. 104, italics in original).

First and foremost, the experience of breast cancer is extremely intimate, private and in many ways specific. The following comment conveys this claim very neatly:

> The most important conclusion for me is that each person's breast cancer is uniquely their own. No two people reach the same medical treatment, nor do any two people with the same diagnosis and survival stats have identical chances of survival. (E-mail 24)

Second, while, as we saw, participants recognize the public dimension of the online spaces in which they participate and publish their stories, they also view these spaces as personal and personalized. The act of expressing their experience in the form of a story, in a space that is seen as highly personalized, invests the story with meanings of uniqueness. The following extract implies the interlink between the personalized character of the online space and the unique value of the postings that are being published in this space:

> After absorbing all of the information garnered from the net and from anecdotal information provided by the "people" genre, I've arrived at several personal conclusions. (E-mail 24)

The "people genre," as the patient in the quote above describes it, contains various discursive forms such as anecdotal information and stories. Patients tend to perceive this "genre"—and thereby the stories that belong to it—as authentic, unique and distinctive. Despite the hundreds of stories published on public online spaces, participants tend to regard them as private and special, particularly in relation to similar stories that are told in mass media, and especially by celebrities who are breast cancer survivors. Patients often associated those mass media stories with negative meanings. Many of my interviewees saw the stories on television as populist, unserious, appealing to the lowest common denominator, misleading and consequently even dangerous, as they might influence women who suffer from the disease to make unreasonable decisions regarding their treatment. In contrast to this public storytelling in mass media, patients usually regard their and their fellow sufferers' disclosure of their experience online as having a clear sense of the private. Storytelling online is seen as intimate, related to a kind of inwardness and subjective experience and appealing to a specific public rather than to the mass public.

However, the distinction between online and mass-mediated storytelling as "private" versus "public" is not that clear-cut. A few of my informants also described patients' stories that they encountered online as "public" in character in the sense of being inauthentic and populist. These kinds of online stories were often associated with a commercial motive. For instance, B (interview 2) describes one of the stories she read in a breast cancer website as a means of "cashing breast cancer," as she puts it. She accuses this kind of online story of negative public characteristics: commercially driven (funded by a medical organization) and thus inauthentic and utilitarian. By the same token, there were also a few references to stories patients heard on television or in magazines as "private" insofar as they were personal, relating a highly subjective experience and told in an intimate fashion.

Interacting Personally, Performing Publicly

Storytelling online is implicated in yet another way in the negotiations between private and public. On the one hand, participants conceive it as an interpersonal, concealed interaction that is restricted to few. On the other hand, it constitutes a performative act that is seen by participants as public and open to all.

Safe Spaces for Private Interaction

Online texts, being disembodied and anonymous, are often seen by patients as confidential and concealed. Online, patients can restrict the distribution of their messages to specific listeners, for instance by using e-mail. Patients seem to appreciate these "private" values, especially in comparison to embodied offline contexts in which their experience is being told. In contrast to online spaces, embodied spaces are open to everyone, in physical view of others. As such, they are beyond the control of the patient:

> It gets me very angry when I hear people know my circumstances whom I didn't tell… If I were a friend of them, I'd [have] told them, but if I'm just acquaintance with them, I didn't, because we don't know each other. So when I found out that they know, I get mad… This is not information to share, no one should know that. It's a very personal thing. (A, Interview 1)

The story of A's illness was circulated through the grapevine. In embodied contexts such as one's offline community, a patient's story can be expropriated from her private realm without her intention or will. In contrast to this kind of space, patients like A perceive online spaces as "safe." They believe that online spaces enable them to restrict the sharing of their personal experience to a specific audience, and to guarantee a level of invisibility within visibility. Illustrative of patients' perception of the online space as private and safe is B's following comment:

> I'm very loud within the breast cancer community, but not in the general public. (Interview 2)

For B, there are clear boundaries between what she considers to be a relatively intimate private space of the "breast cancer community" and that of the "general public." For her, patients' online spaces are part of that "breast cancer community" where she feels comfortable to be "loud." She is a very active participant in various breast cancer-related sites. It is through the delineation of the boundaries of online space as a closed, private community and its distinction from the "general public" that B legitimizes and acknowledges the significance of her online activity, especially storytelling.

Public Performative Spaces

At the same time, patients perceive online spaces also as public venues that possess opposing characteristics: open to everyone, visible and performative. Indicative is patients' awareness of the risk involved in posting their messages in online spaces. Take, for instance, A's following reflection. She clearly acknowledges the inherently public, and thus not hermetically safe, character of online space:

> [S]ometimes it's a little risky to put up yours [story, online], because some people kind of would talk about it. One girl suggested that so and so get in contact with the hospice. Now, I know hospice to be for terminally ill people, and then they were "oh, you know obviously nothing about hospice." Do you understand? She was recommending hospice for someone else, so I said I don't think that's a good idea, because this girl has a hard time coping with breast cancer and you're telling her to contact hospice? [laughs]. (Interview 1)

However, patients' recognition of the open-to-all public dimension of online spaces is not charged only with negative meanings. Some patients refer to their writing in online spaces in terms of a performance, an act that they view in positive terms. "I'm on the board" says B, "it's out there ... it's on 'suite101,' it's on 'Ask Me,'" she comments, referring to her online column. Like B, other patients too relate their act of writing online as a kind of performance before their online readers. They emphasize the influence they have on their "audience." For example, N (e-mail 6) explains her motivation in launching her personal online diary: "people need help, and that is what I'm dedicated to."

The performative dimension of CMC has already been discussed by several scholars in relation to a variety of communicative processes, discursive forms and online contexts (e.g., Chandler, 1998; Paccagnella, 1997; Turkle, 1996; Wynn and Katz, 1997). What seems interesting for the purpose of our discussion is the implication of the performative character of CMC for the act of storytelling. Understanding the work of making a story as a performative act focuses our attention on the interaction between the storyteller and her listeners. More particularly, since their story is to be presented before a particular (although implied and invisible) set of observers, patients want to maintain a continuous presence before their audience. Tellingly, when I approached patients via e-mail, asking them to participate in my study following the messages they had posted in online spaces, respondents would commonly reply asking me to first refer them to their original online posting:

> I shared my stories on several sites and wondered which site that you read my story on? (E-mail 13)

> Please send me the link to shared experience board, I need to review what I had submitted, and I will consider then sharing it with you, there are some updates I am sure since I wrote that. (E-mail 29)

Why did patients ask me to refer them to the "original" story that they posted online? It seems to me that in so doing they try to display coherence and continuity with the story they have performed elsewhere in another online space. The account that they put online constitutes a symbolic "anchor," by which their experience is constructed and organized, and they want to follow this "anchor" with consistency. In this sense, unlike the common view of online narratives as fluid, dynamic and constantly changing (e.g., Hardey, 2002; McLellan, 1997), patients' online accounts seem to represent the opposite. Their circulation in a public space actually endows them with certain fixity. Once a story has transcended the boundaries of a patient's private sphere, or "back region," in Goffman's (1971) terms, extended into the "front region" (i.e., the public sphere of online space), it becomes a publicly available "property" to which the storyteller is committed. She can revisit her story, but she still needs to maintain continuity with the original story she posted.

The need to maintain coherence seems to be particularly emphasized in the context of storytelling, compared to, say, communicating short information on an online message board. This is because a story constitutes a relatively detailed and coherent account that configures a personal experience into a whole and directs it toward some kind of conclusion. Publishing such a discourse seems far more obliging than publishing a short informative text, insofar as it requires the author to maintain the coherence she created, to prolong the "narrative truth" she constructed and to follow up the disclosure that she published in a consistent fashion. This is not to say that patients do not adapt and modify the stories they originally published. Indeed, as I discussed in Chapter 4, the dynamic character of the online communication facilitates an ongoing revision and adaptation of one's personal story. At the same time, there seems to be an amplified performative element that requires the maintenance of consistency, of presenting oneself in a form of a self-narrative rather than using other modes of discourse, which are often more fragmented and less ordered and coherent.

Participants also distinguish between storytelling online as a private act and a performative act that is open to everyone, according to the particular online space in which it takes place. They associate different online venues and environments where they engage in storytelling with a range of meanings, from public and performative to private and intimate. The most important distinction patients make between online spaces is that between message boards and e-mail. While the former is seen as public, the latter is regarded as extremely intimate and private. A good example of this distinction is the way in which both B (interview 2) and G (interview 7) describe occasions in which they moved from communicating on a message board to communicating via e-mail:

> Flora wrote a question to 'Ask Me' [online message board], and I answered her question. She asked me another question, and I said: you know, this is too cumbersome, why don't you just e-mail me direct? She did and then we started talking. (B, interview 2)

> [A]long the way there were a couple of times I got involved with a couple of different women, where we e-mailed one another bypassing the board. (G, interview 7)

It is interesting how G regards the move from the message board (that is, the public space) to e-mail (private space) as an act of "bypassing." For B, too, when the things that are communicated become "too cumbersome," she prefers moving to a one-on-one private mode of communication, namely e-mail. Moving between different online environments is a way of moving between the private and the public, between an intimate interaction and a performance. Of course this is not specific to the act of storytelling, but it nevertheless provides an important context for understanding this activity.

Talking in Experts' and Laypersons' Voices

A fourth aspect of storytelling online, through which patients can negotiate the public and the private in their lives, is associated with the relation between expert and lay knowledge. Warner (2002) identifies this connection: "The epistemological leverage of medical experts ... appears as a very public kind of knowledge and authority, objective and neutral where the patient's claims are understood to be subjective and interested, perhaps even pathological" (p. 53).

However, these classic polarities of "expert" (public) and "lay" (private) are becoming increasingly blurred in online spaces where patients, through the act of writing and narrating their experience, occupy the role of experts, or "semi-experts." Hardey's (2002) and McLellan's (1997) studies of patients' online narratives corroborate this argument, showing how experiential voices take center stage in these narratives.

This phenomenon, however, is not distinctive to the Internet. Recent literature on medical sociology has acknowledged the increasing blurring of boundaries between lay and expert knowledge (Arksey, 1998; Bury, 2001; Lambert and Rose, 1996; Prior, 2003). Health and communication studies in particular highlighted the role of the media in contributing to this process (Hodgetts and Chamberlain, 1999; Seale, 2002). That being said, health representations in the media still largely and mainly serve to support a medical "expert" perspective (Hodgetts and Chamberlain, 1999). Television in particular is a predominantly one-to-many disseminative model of communication. As such, while it gives patients a voice in the public sphere, this voice remains mediated, and crucially framed as private: subjective, experiential, interpretative and informal. Thus, representations of health and illness experiences in the media, especially television, still largely reinforce and reconfirm the lay/expert dichotomy and its respective parallel, the private/public dichotomy.

In contrast to the televisual experience, storytelling online offers patients real opportunities to participate as producers in a public domain, and thus meaningfully challenge the containment of their "private" voice. As I have shown in the previous chapter, by engaging in writing online, especially of a regular column or diary, patients develop a sense of being experts in the subject they write about. B, for example, distinguishes herself from the patient-readers of her online column. She refers to them as "the people" and "the general public," regarding herself as apart from them. Through her engagement in storytelling on a regular online column, she constitutes herself as a "semi-expert" who belongs to a different sphere from that of patients. In so doing she conveys a significant message to herself and her environment, namely: I am a "patient" no longer.

In this sense, patients' online spaces can be seen as spaces for reversal: from lay into expert, from private expression into public discourse. Storytelling is one of the communicative modes through which this reversal is enabled. The form of a personal private story published on an online public forum facilitates the transition from public to private. Therefore, it not surprising that some patients, like K (interview 11) for example, who insist on the maintenance of clear lay/expert private/public boundaries, do not engage in storytelling online, nor in other forms of experiential, lay-to-lay communication online:

> Women are trying to be each other's specialists, advisors when actually they're not in the position to do that. (K, interview 11)

Moving Between the Oral and the Written

The last dimension that I will discuss concerns how storytelling online, in its hybrid oral-written character, provides patients with a mode of communication that helps them craft the boundaries of private and public.

One of the forms that the relation between public and private can take, and which indeed appears central in the context of patients' online communication, is that between the written and the oral. The public is often that which is circulated in print or electronic media, whereas the private is often thought of as circulated orally (Warner, 2002, p. 29). Participants describe their online communication as both oral and written. In the following extracts from patients' accounts, **bolded** text represents references to online communication as "written," whereas *italicized* text represents references to online communication as oral:

> I had two [online] **pen** pals ... if I click with a person, we **correspond** daily.... My friend **writes** me. (E-mail 1)

> We've been *talking* about the World Trade Centre.... She'll [my online pal] *talk* about the length of her hair. And I *told* her [that] chemotherapy changes your hormones.... So she *said*: "Oh, maybe I'll try it." (A, interview 1)

> From "Ask me" [B's online column] I get a lot of questions, a lot of people would also **write** direct. They'd *say* "I saw your name here" ... I have another friend [online pal] ... we were both **posting**, and we started e-mailing ... I've been **corresponding** with her for like three years.... We're not *talking* about breast cancer anymore. Every once in a while we'd *say* "I'm going for my mamo." (B, interview 2)

> I *talk* on a daily basis to 2 other ladies I met on the bcans website.... Even if I don't respond, I still **read** through everyones comments/questions.... Every time I have a doctor apt. [appointment].... All I have to do is get on there [BCANS online forum] and *say* I've got an apt. coming up and I'm overwhelmed with responses and wishes. These ladies have all been where I am now, and got through by *talking* it out with each other. (E-mail 19)

That they use, interchangeably and seamlessly, words that refer to oral and written situations demonstrates the hybrid nature of this communicative situation. On the one hand, the acts of writing (and especially typing), corresponding, posting and reading are acts of literacy. To an extent, they are associated with life contexts that are public, particularly in late modernity. In particular, the online forms into which patients are requested to insert their personal stories often resemble forms that people usually fill out in daily public contexts, for example, financial forms. The instructions of "Shared Experience" website refer to this resemblance directly:

> Add to this Shared Cancer Knowledge
> Please don't think of this as "filling out a form." Be conversational, and write as much as you want, and say whatever you want.

The "Shared Experience" website tells its participants to move away from the public connotation of the act of typing and filling a form, into a private mode of orality: "be **conversational** ... and **say** whatever you want."

On the other hand, this oral conversation has a fundamental literal component. To participate in this conversational situation, one has to express oneself in writing. Recalling Chapter 3, unlike the conventional concept of online conversation, which takes place in a synchronous environment (and is often called "chat," to connote an oral situation), this conversation takes place in an asynchronous environment. As such, it directs participants to textually recount their experience in a coherent way and at length, rather than just chat.

Thus, online communication, and storytelling in particular, offers a special interactional situation consisting of both the written and the oral. The written aspect enables participants to connect the public. Even before an actual dialogic interaction takes place, the act of writing requires the storyteller to step back and dissociate herself from her subjective private sphere, in order to display her story in the public realm—as the following comment captures so well:

> Probably the best part of the internet is that you need to type your question or feeling before you can share it. (E-mail 21)

The oral dimension, on the other hand, emphasizes the private quality of the online interaction. The chattiness enabled by communication via e-mail, or even on message boards, helps participants to delineate their communicative space as private and intimate.

The oral-written hybrid character is emblematic of various other communicative online modes, other than storytelling. Ferrara et al. (1991, in Baym, 2002, p. 65) made a similar claim (however, from a linguistic perspective) about CMC as a hybrid language displaying both oral and written characteristics. More recently, Fernback (2003) has also looked at the enmeshment of the oral and the written in online communication in his examination of discussion groups devoted to urban legends. Relying on Finnegan, who "urges us to move beyond the 'oral' and the 'written' dichotomy" (Fernback, 2003, p. 43), and drawing on earlier studies of CMC, Fernback shows how urban legends circulated in online spaces originate in literate culture (and hence are bound by the structures of literacy), but at the same time exhibit many of the characteristics of oral cultures.

Building upon these works, the analysis presented in this chapter focuses on how the blurred distinctions between the oral and the written, particularly in patients' storytelling online, are connected to negotiations of the public and the private.[43] The following extract from a patient's account of her relationship with her online pal demonstrates this focus:

> I have a dear friend ... who lives somewhere in the State of Wisconsin.... She [We] "type" at each other frequently and I truly feel a bond between us. (E-mail 10)

The bonding between the author and her online pal is the corollary of a hybrid oral-written communicative mode. On the one hand, the author is aware of the significance of the written character of this communication. She chooses the verb "type," to highlight the textual component their relationship is based upon. At the same time, she reflexively puts quotation marks on the word "type," to imply that, in fact, something different is going on here. It is not the regular context of "type" that we might think of, signifying the official, technical, impersonal and, by extension, public. This is, if you wish, an "oral" kind of typing that also entails a "chatty" character: personal, expressive, intimate and, by extension, private. It is the convergence of these seemingly dichotomous characteristics that engenders a genuine bonding between the two patients.

Conclusions: The Dialectical Process of Negotiating Public and Private Online

The terms "private" and "public" often seem to be defined against each other, with normative preference for one term (Warner, 2002, p. 28).

Indeed, the tension between the public and the private and its normative load lurk in much of the debate on individuals' CMC. Most significantly, this tension underlies the debate on the concept of "virtual community" and the concern with the question of whether a genuine community can be sustained through computer-mediated communication. As Bakardjieva (2003) usefully notes, both pessimists and optimists about this question contributed to the framing of the social meaning of the Internet by elaborating the dichotomy between the private and the public:

> Critics like Kumar have seen growing Internet use as contributing to the 'increased privatization and individualization' of existence and the evacuation and diminishing of the public sphere of contemporary western societies' (1995: 163). Enthusiasts, on the other hand, have anticipated invigorated public life and a 'network nation.' (p. 306, citing Hiltz and Turoff, 1978)

As I tried to show in this chapter, patients' practices and experiences of online communication challenge the private/public dichotomy that has framed the discussion of the social meaning of the Internet. Indeed, as Bakardjieva (2003) postulates,

> The preoccupation with ideologically constructed standards, such as virtual community versus real/genuine community and public participation versus privatization of experience, blinds commentators to the possibility of new, unexpected, unimaginable and yet humanist and empowering variations of technological practice to emerge. (p. 311)

Patients' practices reveal a dialectical process of movement between the public and the private. Processes such as storytelling enable the intermeshing of the public and the private in patients' experience. The analysis of these processes, such as the one presented in this chapter, suggests that the values and meanings of public and private should be carefully contextualized. There is no preset preference for the private or the public; their salience to participants' experience differs according to the participants' respective situations, and according to the specific online environment in which they communicate.

Even Bakardjieva, who sensitively recognizes the caveat of framing individuals' use of the Internet in terms of the private/public dichotomy, claiming for the enmeshment of the two in participants' experience falls into the normative trap of regarding the public as normatively superior. The significance of the emerging range of social forms of online communication is not, as Bakardjieva (2003) suggests, unidirectional, "transcending the narrowly private existence" (p. 294) of participants. Rather, the significance of the manifold social forms of online communication is in the ways they enable participants—in this study, breast cancer patients—to negotiate the boundaries of the public and the private in their lives in both directions, back and forth. Negotiating the public and the private, as shown in this chapter, constitutes a key process in patients' endeavor to construct their social reality in a way that would allow them the capacity to act. Storytelling constitutes a key communicative process through which those negotiations take place.

Survival as a Public Testimony

The online scene of breast cancer offers patients a space for public testimony. Online spaces of breast cancer patients constitute collective scenes of disclosure that enable patients to transcend private meanings. Although the display of private matters in those spaces—for example, in the form of self-narratives—is sometimes seen, especially by outsiders, as an erosion of any distinction between public and private, in the actual setting of this communicative space, such displays often have the aim of transformation (Warner, 2002). The visceral intensity of meanings of corporeal pain, shame, guilt, anger and other feelings, and their continual recitation, extend them from the private sphere into the public realm (Warner, 2002). Writing one's experience allows an unspeakable truth to erupt onto the social scene, offering a public testimony. And the therapeutic effect emerges from the individual's capacity to share his/her suffering. The publication of the story (onto the public realm) enables bearing the unbearable (Rosenblum, 2000). Thus, as Stacey (1997) observes, "The stories no longer 'belong to me' but become part of a repertoire of collective narratives of cancer" (p. 242), and as a consequence "Publicness itself has a visceral resonance" (Warner, 2002, p. 63).

As I showed throughout this chapter, by appearing in online interactive forums, a patient's story becomes part of a repertoire of collective narratives of cancer patients. The table displayed earlier, from the "Shared Experience" "online cancer knowledge base," demonstrates this idea eloquently.

Breast Cancer Patients' Online Spaces as Counterpublics

In light of those observations, and with the inspiration of Warner's account of *Publics and Counterpublics* (2002), online sites where patients produce their private accounts can be seen as a collective endeavor that forms a "counterpublic." This counterpublic discursive space does more than represent the interests of breast cancer patients in a public sphere. It mediates the most private and intimate meanings of the experience of illness. In so doing, it works to elaborate new social relations in which the identity of breast cancer patients can be lived, developing its particular forms of association, vocabularies, disembodied practices and relations of camaraderie and communitas. It can make possible new forms of participation in a social world.

Patients' online counterpublic constitutes a scene of association and identity that transforms the private lives it mediates. This counterpublic is not a natural collection of people, nor is it just "community," as Internet researchers would commonly describe it. Closely drawing on Warner's (2002) account of "counterpublics" as mediated publics, breast cancer patients' online participation could be better understood as forming a mediated public rather than a natural community. Like counterpublics of sex and gender, patients' online counterpublics teach us

> to recognize in newer and deeper ways how privacy is publicly constructed. They are testing our understanding of how private life can be made publicly relevant. And they are elaborating not only new shared worlds and critical languages but also new privacies, new individuals, new bodies, new intimacies, and new citizenships. (Warner, 2002, p. 62)

Crucially, as Warner (2002) asserts, counterpublics are embedded in larger publics. The remainder of this chapter focuses on two such contexts, in which breast cancer patients' online communication, and especially the act of storytelling, are embedded. The production and display of patients' self-narratives online, through which, among other processes, patients negotiate the public and private, could not have had a transformative effect if it were not ingrained in a wider cultural and social environment. In this environment, I suggest, two contexts are key: the feminist debate and the culture of the enterprising self (Rose, 1992).

The Feminist Debate

The issue of publicness is intimately interlinked with the feminist debate. The feminist movement has fought against silencing techniques by creating forums where survivors can speak: in magazines, journals, television, support groups, demonstrations and now the Internet. Indeed, the dichotomy between the private and the public has been central to feminist writing and political struggle. The feminist movement sought to reveal the gendering of public and private in order to explain the subordination of women cross-culturally. Female was to private, which meant domestic spaces and functions, whereas male was to public, which referred to contexts in which men spoke and made decisions for the community (Warner, 2002, p. 32, drawing on Rosaldo's infamous essay, 1974). What is more, the gendering of the public and the private has particular resonance in the context of the discourses of breast cancer (see Chapter 3), as much as in relation to the debate on women and technology, and the Internet in particular. Recent discussion amongst feminist critics, both in academia and beyond, revolved around the question of whether computer-mediated communication reinforces or challenges the traditionally gender-associated distinction of private and public.[44]

This is a significant background against which breast cancer patients' negotiation of the private and the public, through online narrating and other communicative processes, should be understood. So, although none of my interviewees referred to the feminist debate in their accounts, it appears a significant backdrop for their active participation in the storytelling of the experience of their illness online. The capacity of online space to furnish a legitimate communicative space for the production and display of patients' personal stories is inextricably embedded in a culture where the slogan "the personal is political" has become a central leitmotif.

The Culture of the Enterprising Self

> Get over your problems, and get off yourself, and work your life! (A, interview 1)

> Become whole, become what you want, become yourself: the individual is to become, as it were, an entrepreneur of itself, seeking to maximize its own powers, its own happiness, its own quality of life. ... On the territory of the therapeutic, the conduct of everyday existence is recast as a series of manageable problems to be understood and resolved by technical adjustments in relation to the norm of the autonomous self aspiring to self-possession and happiness. (Rose, 1992, pp. 150–151)

Patients' negotiation of the boundaries of public and private is interlinked with the wider available discourse of self-governance and the enterprising self. The online space furnishes a space for self-presentation, for confession and introspection. Storytelling is one way of providing patients with a framework to reframe suffering and transform it into mastery. It is necessarily in a culture where breast cancer patients celebrate their personal triumph over the disease publicly, on a public train, that online space can flourish as a space for public testimony.[45] However, while activities such as the Victory train are still seen by many (such as A) as violating the boundaries of privacy, the act of disclosing one's personal experience in a disembodied anonymous space appears widely legitimate, if not desirable.

The discussion has come full circle, linking storytelling online as a process of negotiation of the public and private to the wider contexts within which this activity, and breast cancer in general, are embedded, as discussed in Chapter 3. As we saw, this kind of contextualization is vital, if we are to fully and adequately understand why and how participants engage online to negotiate the private and public in their lives, and why this activity is meaningful. In the next chapter, which concludes the book, I will reflect on storytelling more generally, as a way for thinking about online communication as a socially significant activity.

CHAPTER 7

Conclusions

This book has explored the processes of communication and practices that breast cancer patients engage in on Internet spaces, particularly storytelling. I showed how patients engage in online spaces to construct, or struggle to construct, their self-narratives, how their online participation is partly an attempt to communicate their experience by ordering it in time and gearing it to a closure. My main argument was that patients' storytelling online is a socially meaningful activity that is integral to their process of coping with their illness. Participants' struggle to produce self-disclosure and achieve closure in online spaces is part of their endeavor to transform their existing situation and realize their agency.

This closing chapter evaluates the model I developed throughout the book, namely, storytelling, as a conceptual, analytical and methodological tool for thinking about participants' online activities and experiences. In the first part, I consider the benefits and the limitations of this model for the study of breast cancer patients' CMC, evaluating the merits and drawbacks of the book's focus on studying the *process* of producing discourse, rather than concentrating on the discourse itself.

In the second part of this chapter I put the book into perspective, reviewing the specificity of the study of breast cancer patients' CMC and the broader issues that emerge from the study. First, I consider three particular contexts that need to be borne in mind when evaluating the study and its claims: the culture of breast cancer and therapy, the feminine component and the American aspect. These three contexts facilitate, shape and determine participants' engagement in breast cancer Internet spaces. As I have argued throughout the book, contextualization is vital to researchers' understandings of the phenomena they study.

Second, I discuss the broader issues that emerge from the study and expand the concern with storytelling and breast cancer patients' online communication. In particular, I consider the relationship between the

Internet, communication and agency, and the therapeutic value of CMC, particularly for patients. I also discuss the contribution of this study to the broader debate on CMC and the public/private question.

Thinking About Participants' Online Activity as Storytelling: Usefulness and Limitations

From Text to Process

The research agenda on CMC has given considerable attention to the textual properties of online communication. This book moved away from a mere concern with, and reliance on, the text as the researcher's exclusive source for making sense of participants' online communication by focusing on participants' storytelling as a process. The conversational model, which I discussed in Chapter 2, and which has largely influenced the thinking on CMC, put a lot of emphasis on online texts in explaining participants' interactions and communicative processes. This emphasis was reinforced and supported by employing the Conversation Analysis tradition to study online interactions, the application of traditional discourse analysis to explore online communication contexts, and the impact that linguistic and literary approaches had on the study of CMC. In the context of the study of patients' online participation, Hardey's (2002), McLellan's (1997) and Pitts' (2004) studies are clear examples of this approach. Although written from different perspectives, they all regard the actual texts that patients post online as the key source for understanding participants' online activities and their significance. They therefore rely on these texts as the main, and usually sole, data of their research.

This book's choice to frame participants' online communication as storytelling shifted the focus from the texts that participants produce to the processes of communication in which they engage both behind and on the screen. As I have shown throughout, the concept of storytelling suggests that it is not necessarily and merely the actual texts that participants post online that matter, and that can help us understand what is going on. Thus, relying only on the observable representational level of online activities, that is, texts, is not sufficient to capture the complexity of these activities and to explain their significance. Much more can be learned by attending also to the behind-the-screen process of producing, or attempting to produce, these texts. In this study, "storytelling" provided a model that enabled access to processes taking place behind the screen, and how they correspond (or not) with participation on the screen.

On the Screen and Off the Screen

Storytelling is not a distinctively Internet-based activity. It is a social process that is part of individuals' ongoing self-formation, which manifests itself, among other sites, on the Internet. It is not only about the final product of a narrative but also about the continuous struggle to construct experience in discourse. So exploring participants' engagement in storytelling means also looking at what happens off the screen. Thinking about participants' engagement online as storytelling draws or forces attention towards the manifold practices and activities that emerge around the process, often beyond the observable representational level of online activities.

As we saw, storytelling online encompasses different ways of engagement and disengagement: from posting a story, through lurking to logging off. It pulls our attention to the activity of the teller and also to that of the listener, whose presence (although often implicit, and not synchronous) is crucial for the teller to produce her story. The idea of storytelling as a central practice in participants' online experience demands consideration not only of writing and telling practices but also of reading and listening.

The following excerpt from a breast cancer patient to a mailing list of patients neatly summarizes how varied and multifaceted participants' CMC, and storytelling in particular, can be:

> [I]f you want to ... post as much as you want ... even a lot in one day. If you want to, stay silent and get support without posting. If you want to, stay away for a while and come back. We have some members who come and go. AND wow, some of our members "graduate" and feel they are not in need of support ... if those members want to come back ... they are always welcome.

Staying in the background reading messages, as the poster cited above describes it, can play a significant role in a patient's project to "win this game of survival." Lurking, as discussed in Chapter 5, like other kinds of online activities, can be part of a process in which a participant constructs and tells a certain story about herself to herself and to her environment. Accounting for patients' online communication through the prism of storytelling enabled the inclusion of practices and actions that occur *beyond* the discursive representational space on the screen, and that often remain obscured.

As I mentioned in Chapter 3, storytelling has been recognized in medical practice and cancer care in particular as a tool through which patients can explore and transmit emotional meaning (Carlick and Biley, 2004). Part of the therapeutic value of storytelling is that it makes patients articulate their feelings, even without required feedback (Wagner, 1994, cited in Carlick and Biley, 2004). For researchers, this means that, when they explore the process in its online context, a significant part of what participants do with this medium can actually remain inaccessible. As the following patient reflects, storytelling online can happen far from researchers' reach, and yet have powerful therapeutic effects:

> Probably the best part of the internet is that you need to type your question or feeling before you can share it and sometimes just writing it down is a therapy of its own. (E-mail 21)

Hence, researchers need to think beyond and behind the screen. We need to develop tools to access sites where significant aspects of online communication take place, and which are not accessible through the screen. One such tool, as this quote reveals and as I have shown in this book, is asking participants to reflect on their experience of online participation. Another strategy is an ethnographic approach to the study of Internet communication, as exemplified in the study of Miller and Slater (2000).

In short, the book developed storytelling as a tool to encompass two different settings of Internet culture: "on the screen," that is, observable online texts, in the form of patients' stories, and "behind the screen," that is, processes, activities and practices in which participants engage, that emerge from and around storytelling. This model is an attempt to bridge the two apparently dichotomous and mutually exclusive views of "Internet as culture" and "Internet as cultural artifact." Hine (2000) offered the latter distinction to describe existing common thinking in CMC literature. The first view of "Internet as culture" regards the Internet as a place, a social space in its own right, where culture is formed and reformed. The second perspective, of the "Internet as a cultural artifact," perceives the Internet as a medium. It asks how the Internet is used as a means of communication within users' offline social world. While each of these categories has considerable explanatory power in its own right, as Hine admits, the distinction does not necessarily exist in users' actual experience, nor does it represent a straightforward reflection of online/offline boundary (p. 39).

The model of storytelling enabled this study to encompass the dichotomous distinction conceptually, analytically and methodologically. It showed that the distinction between Internet as culture and Internet as cultural artifact (and thereby between online and offline) does not necessarily exist in breast cancer patients' actual experience. For them, the Internet constitutes both a place and a medium.

Internet as culture. It is evident throughout the analysis that many patients conceive of the Internet as a kind of a place to be. Some described the online context explicitly in terms of a "place," for instance:

> [I]nterpersonal relationships are a vital factor for healing in the /body/mind/spirit connection during the entire process. Doctors who treat a patient like an intelligent fellow human, nurses who are careful and considerate of a weakened body and spirit, medical techs who are empathetic to a patient's fear and frayed nerves, and a support system of close friends and loving family make up the mix that's guaranteed to facilitate healing and peace of mind, provided the patient is herself/himself open to healing. **The internet was the only place**, in the beginning of my bc [breast cancer] journey, where those vital elements were present.... My sanity and peace of mind are a testament to the effectiveness of internet support groups. (E-mail 24, my emphasis)

The Internet appears as a place where patients, among other activities, evaluate their personal stories in relation to those of their peers, consider alternative versions of these stories, refigure their lives in accordance with their chosen version of the stories of which they are part, and consequently take responsibility for their lives. In enabling these processes (which I grouped under the concept of "storytelling"), for breast cancer patients the Internet serves as a place for agency, where they can become creative agents of their experience and identity.[46] The metaphor of a family, which patients often use to describe their belonging to the online space in which they participate, encapsulates their view of the Internet as a self-contained culture within which forms of communication, sociality and identity are produced.

Internet as cultural artifact. At the same time, for some patients, the Internet is not only a place but also a means of communication, embedded in their everyday lives. It is a medium they employ within their existing social world, in order to communicate their experience, often in story form. The transformation through which they go, by participating in storytelling online, is inextricably connected to, and embedded in, their social life. This is unlike the view of the online participant as "the voyager in virtuality" who "return[s] to a real world better equipped to understand its artifices" (Turkle, 1996, p. 263), and for whom the source of the transformation is in the separation between the online and the offline experiences. Here, the transformation for breast cancer patients lies in the inseparability of their online and offline worlds.

In short, as Hine asserts, the distinction between the Internet as culture and as cultural artifact should serve merely as a heuristic device for thinking about the indeterminacy of the Internet. This book's exploration of participants' online activity as storytelling has enabled a complex understanding of the Internet: as a creative and playful place but also as a functional and practical medium, a space in its own right, often perceived by participants as magical and fantastic, but at the same time deeply connected with other spaces and contexts in their lives—the generator of processes, practices and forms of communication, for example, of what I described as "online communitas," and also the product of existing cultures, norms and discourses. Such a combined approach allows a more complex understanding of CMC, identifying its unique and varied qualities, while at the same time recognizing participants' online engagement in continuity with other social practices, and within the wider cultural and social context of their lives.

Storytelling Online as Action

The question of why what we study is important is probably *the* question every researcher grapples with. The argument of this book is that for breast cancer patients the Internet is important because, among other reasons, it constitutes a space and a means to configure their experience into a story. Informed by Ricoeur's theory of storytelling and its developments, I argued that patients' engagement in storytelling online is a way to maintain their capacity to be agents: to have plans and desires, and to hold on to a sense of themselves as agents who have control, however little, over their lives. Through self-narratives that they exchange, patients are able to reach out to each other, help other sufferers and at the same time help themselves, by seeking reassurance and gaining better control over their experience of cancer. Storytelling online is a means in patients' *rite de passage*, releasing them from their previous dominant structure as healthy persons into a liminal phase with fellow sufferers online, to be able "to return to structure revitalized by their experience of communitas" (Turner, 1969, p. 129). I particularly stressed how participants' engagement in storytelling is geared towards their constitution as survivors; how this ongoing activity directs them towards their reincorporation into the "healthy structure." The ongoing struggle to narrate and tell their experience online plays a crucial role in fashioning patients anew, endowing them "with additional powers to enable them to cope with their new station in life" (p. 95).In short, the act of storytelling online is significant because it constitutes an action. Unlike the idea that "the Internet" has certain "effects" or "impact" on its users, the notion of storytelling conceives the "effect" as embedded in the act of storytelling. The hermeneutic approach, which I discussed in Chapter 2, regards the relation between storytelling and agency (or action) as interpretative and cyclical: agency is not only the product of the process of storytelling but also its source. So by engaging in storytelling online—whether by actually producing a story and posting it, or by struggling to produce it, whatever this struggle may entail—participants transform their conditions and realize their agency, however little or limited this transformation may be.

Understanding participants' storytelling online as action challenges a moral problem that arises in individuals' engagement in other media, especially television. Bauman (2001) accounts for this moral challenge:

> [W]hat form can commitment take when those called upon to act are "thousands of miles away from the persons suffering, comfortably installed in front of the television set in the shelter of their homes[?]"47
>
> [W]hile our hands have not grown any longer, we have acquired "artificial eyes" which enable us to see what our own eyes never would. The challenges to our moral conscience exceed many times over that conscience's ability to cope and stand up to challenge. To restore the lost moral balance, we need "artificial hands" stretching as far as our artificial eyes are able to. (p. 2)

This abysmal gap between the suffering that individuals see and their ability to help the sufferers is bridged, to a large extent, in the online communication of breast cancer patients. Unlike reading a personal story of a breast cancer patient in a newspaper, or watching a breast cancer patient's confessional story on television, storytelling online offers direct access to reciprocity with the sufferer. In this sense, patients' online stories provide their creators with "artificial hands," to reach out towards their fellow sufferers. As Susan, a breast cancer survivor, writes to her online protégée, Lara (a fictional e-mail):

> I'm happy to hold your hand until you get the all-clear. (Katz Becker, 2000, p. 13)

Online, participants like Susan and Lara acquire "artificial hands," with which they can meaningfully "hold" each other. They can overcome, at least to some degree, the incapability that Bauman describes, and act upon the suffering they encounter. This is because online, text can constitute a social action; what one writes or says is what one does. Of course, other forms of textual expression online can be equally regarded as actions. The most obvious example in this context is perhaps "cybersex" and the claim that online textuality constitutes sexual action (Slater, 2002, p. 541). Still, unlike other manifestations of online textuality, in storytelling participants employ particular textual "configurational arrangements" (Ricoeur, 1984, p. 67) in an attempt to transform the different events of their experience into a meaningful whole. In particular, the meaning of storytelling as action lies in the storyteller's attempt to impose a sense of ending. It is in this particular act of configuration and closure, unlike in any other online textual activities, that the transformative potency of storytelling lies.

The Limitations of the Model of Storytelling

Yet for all the usefulness of storytelling and its explanatory power as a model for thinking about the social significance of CMC, it suffers from two main limitations.

The difficulty of demonstrating online and offline connections. The idea that participants' storytelling online is a socially significant activity relies on the premise—which I discussed in Chapter 2, drawing primarily on Ricoeur's work—that action exists in the realm of thought and discourse. Thus, the transformative capacity of storytelling exists in the very act of construction and telling the story. In this sense, participants' engagement in storytelling online is an act that intermeshes the online and offline, insofar as it takes place online, but at the same time can transform participants' (offline) behavior and feelings in meaningful ways.

However, those who think of action as occurring beyond the realm of thought and discourse would not accept so easily the idea that storytelling online is necessarily a process intermeshing participants' online and offline worlds. For them, the key concern would be the extent to which participants' storytelling online indeed translates into action in other realms of everyday life. This line of thinking, as I mentioned in Chapter 2, would have produced a very different kind of study: one that would examine other actions and constructions, beyond those of participants' storytelling online, and try to draw the connections (and possibly also disconnections) between them and participants' online experience.

I accept the claim that patients' storytelling online may represent their intentions and desires, but not necessarily correspond with their actual capacity to fulfill these desires, that is, with their capability to act beyond the realm of the story they tell. And that without exhaustive ethnographic or other kinds of data we cannot reveal such contradictions between what participants do online and what they do, or do not do, offline. There was a strong sense of empowerment and, at times, even omnipotence, that emerged from participants' accounts about their online participation and its significance. It might be that if I had studied patients' lives ethnographically—say, by observing other activities in their lives across time—their online participation would have appeared less empowering, and perhaps even disempowering. It might be that more disconnections and contradiction between their online experiences and offline contexts would have emerged.

I do think, nevertheless, that the sense of storytelling online as curative and therapeutic, and more generally the sense of being able to transform one's life and cure oneself through talking, is a coin of the very phenomenon that I studied. In other words, the utopian sense that emerges from the data—participants' online and face-to-face accounts, as well as website texts—cannot be simply dismissed as a limited account of patients' online experience, which is disconnected from, or unsupported by, offline "evidence." Rather, the way patients describe their online participation as largely empowering, therapeutic and "cheerful" is indeed a key characteristic of this communicative context.[48] Storytelling of breast cancer patients on the Internet is about the capacity to act, rather than about the failure to do so.

The difficulty of distinguishing storytelling from other online activities. The move from a concern with the textual properties of online communication to a focus on participants' engagement in the process of storytelling runs the risk of ending up with a very broad analysis. Since storytelling, unlike "online narratives," is not anchored by a clear delimited textual form, but rather refers to the process of production or the struggle to produce this text, it can easily become a vague concept that encompasses too many things. In particular, throughout the analysis, it was often difficult to draw the boundaries between "writing" and "storytelling." Clearly, not every time a patient writes something online does she engage in storytelling. But to determine that the communicative activity at stake is storytelling, rather than simply writing, we need to look for specific textual properties.

Similarly, it is often hard to distinguish storytelling from the broader process of sense making and self-disclosure. Storytelling is only one particular process by which sense making and self-disclosure are exercised and performed. The theoretical assertion that underlined my inquiry was that individuals understand themselves and construct their self-identity by working and reworking their interpretation of their own biography in the form of a narrative and a story (Giddens, 1991; Thompson, 1995). Further, since my analysis did not focus on the final product of this process, that is, the discursive form of narrative, but on the act of construction, interpretation and reinterpretation, demarcating what counts as storytelling and what counts as sense making has sometimes been tricky.

In attempting to address these difficulties, throughout the book I aimed to clarify and qualify the specificity of storytelling, particularly by drawing on Ricoeur's theorization, and emphasizing storytelling as an attempt to configure events in temporal order and direct them toward closure. Nevertheless, I admit that distinguishing this process from other related categories, such as writing or sense making, remains difficult. This difficulty, however, is not limited to the attempt to apply the concept to the online context of breast cancer patients. It seems to me that it is a broader conceptual pitfall of the theory of narrating and storytelling. When it is understood as the fundamental process of experiencing time, storytelling gains a very central, if not a ubiquitous, status in social life. So it often appears to be an all-embracing process.[49]

Despite this difficulty, my aim has been to show how describing patients' online participation as a process of storytelling can illuminate the specific processes of communication and Internet spaces in which they engage, in ways that other models would not have been able to. In particular, understanding patients' online activity as storytelling showed that their online communication does not center only on information seeking, an aspect with which the "e-health" literature has been quite preoccupied. It also helped specify the particular aspects and social consequences of what has been often explained in general terms such as "emotional support," "esteem support" (Shaw et al., 2000), "social support" (Sharf, 1997) and "empowerment" (Pitts, 2004; Sharf, 1997). It stressed that what participants do online is part of their engagement in a broader process of self-formation and self-elaboration, of coping with a disease and reworking their identity.

This is not to suggest that participants, and patients in particular, do not and cannot engage in "one-off" activities online, such as what B describes:

> Some people also wanted just to ask their questions, and they would discuss their subjects again. Get your information, and then they want no connection. (Interview 2)

Arguably, this kind of immediate, short-term, information-oriented participation constitutes a significant part of patients' online activity. Yet it does not necessarily have to do with a complex process of identity construction through an attempt to configure experience and direct it toward closure. This kind of more practical and even instrumental activity has been widely studied in what I described as the information-seeking paradigm. Storytelling should therefore be seen as a model that complements, rather than contradicts or supersedes, other models that account for participants' online activities.

The Scope of the Book

The book examined a specific health context in which CMC takes place, namely breast cancer. In doing so, it lays claim to being a contribution to understanding the ways in which meanings of health, and breast cancer in particular, are constructed and negotiated via patients' online participation. Although I have used the case of the online communication of breast cancer patients to understand broader aspects of CMC, it is important to bear in mind that the practices, relations and processes described in this study, and particularly the act of storytelling, emerge in a particular setting and a particular context.

The Culture of Breast Cancer and Therapy

First, the phenomenon of self-disclosure and the centrality of storytelling are closely embedded within the cultures of breast cancer, and of therapy and self-help, which emphasize these practices (as discussed in

Chapter 3). Arguably, these practices would take quite a different shape, volume and style in other contexts communicated online. This point reinforces, of course, the inseparability of online and offline in examining CMC. In other words, the contexts within which the phenomenon studied here is embedded are pivotal in order to get to grips with its online and offline social meanings.

Second, the exchange-based relations that develop and are maintained online between breast cancer patients are also significantly set in a specific social and cultural context of breast cancer, a context that allows and perpetuates this kind of relationship. A look at health-related public interactive forums, where patients exchange experiences, reveals the prominence of breast cancer over other health contexts, including other types of chronic illness. This does not mean that exchange relations do not occupy a central role in other health as much as non-health online environments. Indeed, studies such as Preece and Ghozati's (2001) have shown the centrality of exchange in a different health-related context of online communication, namely, knee injuries. Other authors (e.g., Kollock, 1999) acknowledged exchange as key to the relationships that emerge between participants online in non-health contexts. However, bearing in mind that exchange relations are a general feature of CMC, in examining a specific online landscape such as that of breast cancer patients, we should also account for the significance of the particular communicative and cultural environment of breast cancer and therapy, that allows, encourages and legitimizes this aspect of communication between patients.

Third, although the private/public issue that was discussed in Chapter 6 has much to suggest beyond the specific context of breast cancer CMC, nevertheless it has a clear component that stems from the particular nature of breast cancer and its social construction. Arguably, more than many other experiences being communicated online, even if those are health-related, breast cancer evokes an inescapable tension between the private and the public, regardless of CMC. Breast cancer is a highly intimate experience, whose social construction is imbued with meanings of publicity, publicness and, by extension, "publishing the self" (Potts, 2000). So whereas similar tensions probably arise in other CMC contexts, I think that the centrality of these tensions in this study is greatly influenced by the actual content and context of the communication under scrutiny.

The Feminine Component

Another specific aspect of breast cancer patients' online communication is its feminine bias. Breast cancer CMC is a communicative context on a women's issue, by women and for women. The online communication of breast cancer is predominantly female because the disease is overwhelmingly a women's illness. In addition, statistics consistently document that women constitute the main seekers of information on health online (Datamonitor, 2002; Houston and Allison, 2002; Pew Internet & American Life, 2002a, 2003).

So some, including two of my interviewees, might argue that the fact that it is such a women-based communication determines its features in significant ways—for instance, that the centrality of practices and relations of exchange, bonding and self-disclosure has to do largely with the femininity of this communication. This aspect, however, was not developed in this study. The unit of analysis of this study was not women who suffer from breast cancer and participate in related Internet spaces, but rather the process of storytelling in online spaces. In my examination of breast cancer patients' online engagement, primarily on the basis of participants' accounts, the gender of the participants seemed to be only one factor, among many others, that frames their online experience. So, the study aimed to map out the key dimensions of this experience, accounting for the gender aspect only when it was empirically relevant. It would be interesting for future research to account for this aspect. Pitts (2004), for example, has explored some aspects of breast cancer patients' web pages, highlighting some gender-specific issues that characterize these communicative spaces.

The Cultural Specificity of CMC

The online communication of breast cancer patients occurs within a certain cultural setting that shapes their communicative spaces in significant ways. As with the feminine aspect, this book has not discussed the cultural dimension so far. It is outside the scope of this book to tackle this aspect in depth and I develop it in greater length elsewhere (Orgad, 2006). However, the matter deserves some attention here so that the issues raised in this book will be seen in perspective. Given the available space, my aim here is to present only preliminary thoughts to stimulate further discussion in relation to the study of the cultural specificity of CMC.

When I started the investigation of the online communication of breast cancer patients, I thought about the Internet in terms of a universal, nonspecific communicative space that was undifferentiated by cultural or national boundaries. Clearly, I was influenced by the view that seemed to have overwhelmed the debate at the time, in academia and beyond, of the Internet as a borderless space. Most of the discussion of health-related CMC seemed to particularly enhance this view, regarding users' experience as essentially boundless in terms of its cultural context (e.g., Hardey, 2002). At face value, breast cancer patients' Internet spaces seemed to constitute borderless and cultureless sites, where patients communicate a universal disease across the globe, beyond geographical, cultural or national boundaries.

To a certain extent, this is indeed true. There is a strong sense of commonality and universality that emerges between participants on these spaces, as I emphasized in Chapter 5. Women from various cultural backgrounds participate in these sites, although there is no consistent data that confirms this observation. The concept of storytelling as a central communicative mode endorsed the idea of the borderless nature of patients' CMC. Storytelling is a universal communicative process that arguably enables patients to develop communication that occurs beyond cultural or other boundaries. Furthermore, participants themselves seemed to subscribe to a view of the Internet as borderless and globally inclusive. My interviewees often stressed how by posting their message online they reached out to patients who are remote from their locale, geographically and/or culturally. Participants tended to see reaching readers on a worldwide scale as a sign that their messages have meaningful value, beyond their personal, locally bound realm.

However, I suggest that the online communication of breast cancer patients takes place within cultural settings that have significant North American resonance. Although they are often invisible, there are certain cultural elements that underlie breast cancer patients' online communication. They provide specific forms of language, clichés, motifs, references and other symbolic repertoires that allow and constrain what is said (and what is not), and how it is expressed on patients' Internet spaces. These elements, I argue, are to a large extent North American. In particular, the proliferation of patients' personal online stories of survivorship, which I demonstrated throughout the book, is closely related to the American context, within which these stories are constructed and told.

In suggesting that breast cancer patients' CMC has significant North American resonance, by no means do I mean to imply that "North American culture" is a homogenous, monolithic entity. I do, however, suggest that there are certain values, symbols, discourses and beliefs that are characteristic of what a person in North America, and particularly the United States, is socialized by and acculturated to, that underpin the communicative context of breast cancer online.

To start with, the majority of respondents to my online recruitment message were from the United States. Recruiting non-American respondents proved very difficult, although I deliberately tried to avoid posting my message on national websites such as that of the American Cancer Society. Later, I also tried to specifically recruit women from the United Kingdom by posting messages on U.K. websites. Remarkably, however, I hardly received any replies whereas messages I posted on ".com" or ".org" sites had generated several, usually from North American respondents.

Arguably, that I used English search terms, and posted a recruitment message in English, biased my sample to English-speaking participants. Another possible explanation for the American bias is, of course, that more American breast cancer patients are connected than other patients in the world. Still, I do not think it is coincidental that the majority of the mainly English-speaking respondents were American.

I suggest that the willingness to disclose one's personal experience has to do with the American context of those respondents. The idea that "If you talk about something you feel, then you will feel better" and the almost religious belief in the power of language to facilitate change is characteristic of U.S. culture (Polanyi, 1985, p. 146). So the link I presented in this book between storytelling online and the therapeutic is not culturally naked. Rather, this link becomes meaningful within a very specific cultural framework that is underpinned by the idea that it is possible to understand anything and explain it, especially through narrative (Becker, 1994). This framework, I propose, has a significant American imprint. Denzin's (1999) observation reinforces this point: "We cannot imagine America without its self-help groups. And, we cannot imagine an America that is not in love with technology. Cyberspace and the recovery movement were meant for each other" (p. 113).

It is in light of this recognition, of the inextricable link between self-help and particularly the idea of "the talking cure," CMC and U.S. culture, that we can fully and adequately account for what is going on in breast cancer Internet spaces. For instance, by recognizing the American fascination with self-help and CMC, we can fully make sense of comments of the following kind, made by a breast cancer patient who is an active participant in patients' forums:

> The ones who stick around are the fighters ... those that come on and are passive and feel it's just too hard to fight it, give up and give in to their disease and don't stick around. (E-mail 15)

This view of the "fighter" who communicates and "sticks around," versus the "loser" whose logging off from online forums represents her "losing of the battle," is underpinned by an ideological premise that is embedded in an American belief system. It is the ideology of autonomy and self-determination; the idea that the individual is the central figure on the stage of the world (Polanyi, 1985). This cultural myth is one way in which the online and the offline interweave in participants' experience; giving up online is an admittance of giving up offline and vice versa.

Frank (1995) further develops the discussion of the cultural context of this ideology: "North Americans," he says, "share a cultural reluctance to say that their lives have gone badly in some significant respect and to mourn the loss of what was desired but will never happen" (p. 63). Indeed, a reluctance to admit failure and loss seems to be perpetuated in the CMC of breast cancer patients. Key motifs of patients' online discussion are the notable absence of death and the ways in which expressions of despair and hopelessness are being excluded or contained in the postings. The titles of the messages women post, often of painful and difficult experiences, are mostly cheerful and triumphal: "a sense of humor helps," "don't fear having a breast biopsy," "I made it through biopsy without a hitch!" "against all odds," "bald and proud" and "living for love," to mention just a few. The actual content of the messages follows similar lines. The online colloquy of breast cancer is about enablement and hope, as Pitts (2004) and Sharf (1997) showed in their studies; participants make the online discussion about living with the illness, rather than dying from it (Sharf, 1997).

On a more general note, whether the participants are Americans or not, the actual communication in which they are engaged has American underpinnings. They therefore have to work within this setting, which determines what is said and what is not. There are certain "hidden rules," as one of my non-American interviewees described it, that participants have to follow if they are to comfortably engage in the discussions.

This observation suggests that participants should not only be competent in CMC in the technical sense but also have social and cultural competency, that is, knowledge of the discursive frameworks and the "hidden rules" of the communicative context. K, one of the only non-American breast cancer patients whom I interviewed, is perhaps the most computer literate of all my interviewees. However, in a sense, she was not sufficiently culturally competent to participate actively in any of the online discussions. A more complex concept of media literacy is thus desirable, one that involves not only technical knowledge and skill but also cultural competence. This study merely scratches the surface of this potentially rich discussion of the need to expand the concept of Internet literacy.

The point about the cultural specificity of breast cancer patients' CMC also urges an expansion of the research agenda in relation to processes of exclusion and inclusion in CMC. To date, the only literature that has probably engaged with this issue from a cultural perspective is the debate around the digital divide. It questioned the extent to which the online space is indeed inclusive and egalitarian, focusing on the disparities between the "haves" and "have-nots." It accounted for the sociodemographic (and chiefly economic) reasons underlying dynamics of inclusion in and exclusion from online communication. This study calls for the need to include also a critical consideration of the cultural specificity that frames online communicative contexts, and works to exclude and to include certain meanings.

We must also recognize that research methodology has social and cultural borders. It would be naïve to think that doing Internet research means doing borderless or cultureless research. In this study, the search engines I used, the terms I used to search breast cancer websites and the actual websites I visited are not culturally naked, so they informed my study and its findings in significant ways. The methodology employed was also significantly informed by the specificity of participants' cultural location, which facilitated their online recruitment and their collaboration in being interviewed both online and face-to-face. The respondents' openness and the ease with which they very quickly disclosed their intimate experience, is largely due to their U.S. cultural context. A valid question remains: Would I have been able to pursue the same methodology in a different culture with the same degree of success? The answer is "no," at least not in the United Kingdom, if the words of my only British interviewee are anything to go by. "You would have never found me online," she told me.

As much as participants' online experience is fundamentally embedded in their cultural and social context, so are the studies done on them. The contexts of Internet use being examined by organizations such as "Pew Internet & American Life," the methodology employed and the approaches taken are fundamentally North American. This kind of significant research, which determines the research agenda and shapes the way CMC is understood, should be more reflective of the cultural framework in which it is embedded.

All that being said, the recognition of the cultural specificity of breast cancer online communication, its feminine bias and its embeddedness in the culture of breast cancer and therapy, does not disqualify the study's contribution to, and implications for, the wider thinking about CMC. Despite its distinctive aspects, the case of the online communication of breast cancer raises several key issues and broader questions that invite further research. This is the concern of the remainder of this chapter.

Internet, Communication and Agency

The exploration of breast cancer patients' CMC is, more generally, a study of individuals' participation in Internet spaces as a way of realizing their agency. It connects to the broader concern with CMC and its role in people's lives, particularly its potential significance for processes of self-formation and for individuals' elaboration of their self-understanding, not only in situations of crisis such as chronic illness.

So beyond its specific characteristics, the communicative context of breast cancer online provided a scene for examination of the broader concern with the relation between individuals' online communication and processes of agency. The CMC of breast cancer patients constitutes a "magnifying glass" revealing complex connections between participants' online communication and the management of their everyday experiences. It illuminates the Internet as a key communicative space where participants can explore and transmit their feelings and experiences and can appropriate a disembodied medium as a way to transform their life circumstances, however limited the transformation.

The therapeutic value of CMC. More specifically, this study shows that the Internet can act as a meaningful therapeutic site, where participants engage in self-reflexivity and self-interrogation. Significantly, however, the Internet is not inherently a reflexive and therapeutic medium. It is the constellation of the specific ways individuals such as breast cancer patients participate in online spaces, and the particular social and cultural context in which their participation is embedded, that makes the Internet a significant therapeutic space, and that makes storytelling specifically enabling in this respect. The particular social and cultural meanings of breast cancer, especially the stress on patients' need to communicate their experience in the public realm, provide a vital context for the Internet to develop as a key communicative site for breast cancer patients. Equally, the sociotechnical properties of the Internet provide a fruitful setting for the proliferation of breast cancer-related online colloquy, and particularly for patients' appropriation of the new medium for storytelling.

The therapeutic, however, is not unique to the online culture. As I discussed in Chapter 3, it is a central component of wider contemporary culture: communicative spaces where therapeutic practices and processes of self-understanding and self-interrogation are exercised are increasingly expanding. What is significant, then, specifically about the Internet as a therapeutic space?

One of the important things CMC seems to do is to legitimize self-reflection and the performance of the self. By enabling individuals to disclose their experience in a joint-action with other peers, therapeutic practices are being externalized and expropriated from delineated professional spaces of therapy, such as the analyst's couch, into the new communicative space of the Internet. In so doing, the therapeutic becomes an accessible popular "product," rather than something restricted to professional interaction. In this sense, the Internet should be seen as part of a wider contemporary media culture, in which therapy and psychoanalysis are being increasingly popularized. This trend is most associated with audience discussion television programs such as *Jerry Springer* or *Oprah* (see Peck, 1996). Indeed, patients often referred to their Internet activities as related to other mediated therapeutic forms, such as reading self-help books, or watching talk shows about breast cancer experience.

At the same time, CMC seems to embody also different kinds of therapeutic practices and relations from those offered by television audience discussion programs or self-help books. Particularly salient is the different role and power of expertise in the therapeutic space of CMC. Mediated therapeutic forms such as audience discussion television programs are based on the traditional contrast between "lay" and "expert"; they are embedded in a culture that binds us to the power of expertise (Livingstone and Lunt, 1994; Rose, 1992). CMC, as I have shown in the case of breast cancer patients, seems to offer a far more hybrid space, where the boundaries between expert and lay are essentially blurred. This hybrid character of CMC offers a kind of release from the dependence on expertise. First, breast cancer online communicative spaces are designated in a way that excludes experts and intends to include only patients. Second, even if a kind of hierarchy is created among patients, in which some patients take on the role of experts who mentor newcomers, patients' expertise remains contained; they are still, at the end of the day, laypersons. In most of the interviews I conducted it was clear that patients regard online communication with fellow sufferers in very different terms from their communication with their doctors. While there is a clear sense of dependence on the medical experts in their lives, in their online communication patients seem to be released from this reliance on expertise.

However, that patients may appropriate the new opportunities for communication offered by CMC does not necessarily mean that they stop trusting, or even tend to trust less, the experts in their lives. On the contrary, most of the patients I interviewed seem to maintain conventional norms regarding expertise and their trust in experts. Notwithstanding the hybrid lay/expert character of CMC, for most of the patients I interviewed, expertise remains the territory of medical professionals, and is usually associated with offline times and spaces of their medical encounters. Online, on the other hand, is primarily the terrain of "the people genre" (as one of my interviewees called it), that is, a space oriented for the communication of personal experience. And storytelling is one of the ways through which personal experience is communicated.

Thus, online, the therapeutic is promoted and mediated mainly through experiential communication between laypersons, rather than through expert-lay relations. This observation limits, I suggest, the moral panic about the danger of patients being misled by information they get from other laypersons online. It also challenges research such as Stone's infamous study of "The Cross-dressing Psychiatrist" (1995) that stresses the seductiveness of disembodiment and anonymity, and the way participants can be deceived by it. This study shows that online participants are not "dopes" who follow whatever they read online, enchanted by the new opportunities of disembodiment and anonymity; nor do they subscribe that easily and quickly to new forms of knowledge and relationship. Rather, while they embrace new forms of communication and opportunities for voicing their experience, they also maintain conventional thinking about the role and value of expert versus lay knowledge.

Online Communication and the Public/Private Question

Another broader issue that emerges from the study and expands the concern with storytelling and breast cancer patients' online communication relates to the question of "public" versus "private" in CMC. The separation between "private" and "public" has had a strong imprint on the ways CMC has been studied, both in an ontological sense (i.e., the claims made about the essence of CMC) and also regarding methodological and ethical consideration of CMC. A common ontological claim made by Internet scholars has been that online space is a private space, separate from clear "public" spaces. Participants, so the argument goes, perceive what they do and post online as private and restricted to a specific audience. Therefore, the methodological and ethical implication is that researchers should not use any online personal material without participants' consent. Yet other researchers tend to see online environments as public spaces (e.g., Barnes, 2004; Clegg Smith, 2004[50]). They tend to operate with an assumption that informed consent is not required and that disclosing information such as participants' screen names or e-mail addresses is permissible because the information is already publicly available (Chen, Hall and Johns, 2004).

This book sheds a critical light on the private/public distinction that has governed the study on CMC. It suggests that the separation between the public and the private is unsustainable on ontological or ethical grounds. Patients' online spaces, as I argued throughout the book and stressed especially in Chapter 6, form scenes of association that transform the private lives they mediate. In these communicative spaces, rather than acting out a clear-cut separation between private and public, participants continuously negotiate between the two. Participants in online discussions of the extremely intimate and private experience of breast cancer often had a very ambivalent perception of the extent to which their online communication is indeed "private." Thus, generalizations of the kind made by Barnes (2004), that "Often people who are corresponding in public chatrooms or discussion groups perceive their conversation to take place in a private setting" (p. 220), need careful substantiation. In my study, for example, some participants considered online spaces to represent precisely the opposite: a public setting, where their aim is to yield as large and as far reaching a range of responses as possible.

So we cannot simply assume that "online = private." Similarly, we cannot unproblematically work with the assumption that online interactions occur within the public domain, and as such are simply open to general scrutiny (Clegg Smith, 2004, p. 230). Rather, we should inquire into the ways in which meanings of "public" and "private" are constructed online in specific situated contexts, explore the ambiguities that they generate, and consider carefully their implications for research practice. Clearly, while researchers need to make every effort to maintain participants' confidentiality and anonymity, rigid guidelines that do not allow any use of individuals' online communication without participants' consent appear unreasonably restrictive of research and are thus unhelpful. Similarly, an approach underlined by the simplistic assumption that the online space is public, and thus accessible to researchers with no restriction, runs the risk of generating research that has shaky ethical foundations. The key to approaching the private/public question when conducting Internet research is to ground our decisions empirically. In doing so, researchers can "make a more substantive contribution to our understanding than any amount of argument or counterargument could ever accomplish" (Bruckman, 2004, p. 103).

Closure

Every story needs a closure. In closing this book, I want to recall Walter Benjamin's lamenting of the end of the art of storytelling in his seminal essay *The Storyteller*, more than three decades ago (1970). The fading away of storytelling, and thereby of the communicability of experience, Benjamin argued, lies in the rise of a new form of communication: information. The media (for Benjamin, principally the press) are central in this process: everything is now communicated to us, the listeners, in a form of explanation (see also Silverstone, 1999, pp. 40–41). Consequently, "the securest among our possessions were taken from us: the ability to exchange experience" (Benjamin, 1970, p. 83).

This book has shown that Benjamin's assessment was wrong. Storytelling has not come to an end. On the contrary, the Internet, which is often associated with the age of information, facilitates a different kind of communication: the ability to exchange experience, in the form of storytelling. Storytelling online has novel and distinctive qualities, but it is also similar in many ways to the "good old" storytelling that Benjamin is nostalgic about.

Yet in his characterization of the storyteller, I believe Benjamin to have been right. "The storyteller," Benjamin (1970) observes, "is a man who has counsel for his readers.... After all, counsel is less an answer to a question than a proposal concerning the continuation of a story which is just unfolding" (p. 86). The story of the Internet and its role in people's lives is constantly unfolding. It is my hope that this book has offered some counsel to its readers. Rather than giving definite answers or solving issues once and for all, this book is a proposal that will, I hope, contribute to the developing exploration of the Internet in everyday life.

Appendix 1

Sociodemographic Table of Participants

Face-to-face interview		Online narrative	Age	Place of residence	Socio-economic group	Education	Marital status	Children
Name	Inter view				A=high B=middle C=low			
A	1	1	32	suburb, NY, US	A–B	high school	married	none
B	2	2	52	suburb, NY, US	B	BA	married	3
C	3	-	76	suburb, NY, US	B	high school	married	2
D	4	4	50	suburb, NY, US	A–B	MS	married	1
E (man)	5	5	50s	city, NY, US	B	BA	married	none
F	6	-	58	rural area, Connecticut, US	A–B	high school and secretarial school	married (second time)	2
G**	7	-	43	small town, NY, US	B	MS	married	2
H	8	-	65	suburb, New Jersey, US	A–B	BA	married	2 (adopted)
I	9	-	69	suburb, New Jersey, US	A–B	BA	married	2
J	10	-	44	town, New Jersey, US	B	BA	married	2
K	11	-	49	city, UK	B	PhD in progress	married	3
L	12	-	53	town, Israel	A–B	high school	widow	2
(Letter narrative)		3	40	city, Israel	B	BA	married	2
-		6	56	city, Texas, US	B	BA, MS in progress	divorced	5
-		7	43	town, NY, US	B	high school	married	none
-		8***	39	town, NY, US	A–B	BA	married	2
-		9	****	city, UK	B	****	****	****
-		10	58	town, Michigan, US	B	high school and religion studies	married	2
-		11	****	town, NY, US	****	****	married	1
-		12	****	city, Minnesota, US	B	BA	****	****
-		13	40s	city, Texas, US	B	1 year of college	married	none
-		14	52	city, Nevada, US	A	BA	divorced	1
-		15	49	city, California,US	****	****	married	5
-		16	****	city, Washington, US	B	****	*****	*****
-		17	42	city, Greece	B	university	married	none
-		18	48	city, Florida, US	B	high school	married	2
-		19	40s	town, Pennsylvania,US	B	high school	married	2
-		20	50s	city, Missouri, US	B	****	married	5
-		21	****	town, North Dakota, US	****	****	married	****
-		22	****	rural area, Oregon, US	****	****	married	none
-		23	****	small town, Georgia, US	****	****	married	no. not specified
-		24	50s	town, Virginia, US	B	university	married twice	2
-		25	50s	rural area, Michigan, US	B	high school	married	3
-		26	48	small town, Louisiana, US	B	high school	married	2
-		27	40s	city, Florida, US	B	****	****	****
-		28	42	small city, Arkansas, US	B	****	****	****
-		29	42	city, NY, US	B	****	married	no. not specified

See legend on next page

* The details were correct at the time when the participants took part in the study (face-to-face interviews: time of interview; online narratives: time of writing the account).

** Telephone interview.

*** The patient in narrative 8 was supposed to meet me for a face-to-face interview; however, the interview was cancelled at the last moment following deterioration in her health.

**** Data missing.

Notes

1. http://www.sharedexperience.org
2. http://www.acscsn.org/Forum/Discussion/summary.html
3. A similar experience was indicated by the researchers of Pew Internet & American Life (2003), where interviewees were sent a semistructured questionnaire about their health-related Internet use. Rather than following the question-and-answer format, respondents elaborated about their personal stories.
4. This reflection is based on Bauer and Gaskell (2000, p. 39).
5. See the Association of Internet Researchers' ethics recommendations: www.aoir.org/reports/ethics.pdf
6. The studies of Pew Internet & American Life refer to American users who seek health information online. Some studies claim that Americans are significantly more likely than Europeans to do this (Goldstein, 2003). I address the cultural aspect of Internet use in the concluding chapter.
7. The only study I came across that provides a consistent account of the issue is *Hamlet on the Holodeck: The Future of Narrative in Cyberspace* (Murray, 1998). This study provides useful insights into the ways in which computer-mediated communication both changes and shapes narratives and stories. It is limited, however, particularly compared with the approach in my study in two main respects. Firstly, its focus is on narratives rather than narrating. It is written from a literary perspective, examining what happens to narratives when they move from classic formats (e.g., novels) into computer-mediated forms. Secondly, Murray's analysis is primarily concerned with digital environments of interactive fiction: stories in which participants engage in role-playing, interacting with automated characters on imagined online landscapes. In this sense, it aligns itself, to a large extent, with other studies that focus on notions such as disembodiment and virtuality, a focus of which this book is highly critical.
8. For example, the issue of the *Journal of Computer-Mediated Communication* entitled "Persistent Conversation" presents a collection of essays concerning online conversation. However, there seems to be a very weak link between the different definitions and perspectives of online conversation that are suggested in the different essays. Consequently, online conversation seems to have too many meanings, with no clear reference.
9. In this study, the notions of "narrative" and "story" are often used interchangeably. It should be noted, however, that in some schools of narrative analysis, the terms have come to designate two quite distinct phenomena; narrative often refers to discursive rendering, whereas "story" refers to the underlying events that the narrative recounts (Mattingly and Garro, 2000, p. 12).
10. Although I use Silverstone's work here to exemplify a structuralist narrative analysis of media texts, it should be noted that Silverstone's approach is not purely structuralist. Rather, in his work, Silverstone (1988, 1994) combines an acknowledgment of the structural elements of television, with a view of media consumers as crucially engaged in interpretative processes.
11. I develop this point elsewhere; see Orgad, 2005b.

12. During the nineteenth century, women supposedly accounted for three-fifths of all cancer cases (Lerner, 2001, p. 46).
13. See Hydén (1997) for a comprehensive review of how social scientific studies of illness and biomedical studies have made use of the narrative concept.
14. www.dipex.org
15. www.expertpatients.nhs.uk
16. White (1980) claims that, in the historical documents he examines, the representation of events in the form of annals is a conscious and purposive "refusal to narrate" (p. 14) on the part of the annalist.
17. www.sharedexperience.org
18. See for example, www.breastcancer.org, "Biographies of breast cancer survivors" message board and www.breastcancergroup.org/ourstories.html.
19. e.g., www.oncochat.org
20. The URL is www.sharedexperience.org. At the time of writing, this text had been recently removed.
21. In this respect, the face-to-face interviews were crucial insofar as they exposed the centrality of the online experience in patients' coping; in their online accounts, the same interviewees dismissed the role of the Internet in their coping.
22. This is the only written account that was sent to me as a letter in the post and not as e-mail.
23. www.sharedexperinece.org/experienceadd.lasso
24. The BCANS message board is divided into "on-topic" and "off-topic" boards. I explain this later.
25. http://bcans.ca/forum/help.htm
26. This view echoes the emphasis on the constructive nature of reading in literary theory and the notion of the "active viewer" in media audience studies, by which the reader/viewer is seen as actively engaging in the interpretation of the text, despite her apparent passivity.
27. www.bcans.org
28. The linkage between liminality, communitas and storytelling loosely evokes Turner's observation that liminality is a condition in which myths and symbols are frequently generated (Turner, 1969, p. 128).
29. The original authors' names have been changed.
30. http://bca.ns.ca/booklets/inourown.pdf
31. See endnote 30.
32. This message has been significantly led by feminist forces embedded in organizations such as the (American) National Breast Cancer Coalition (NABCO) (Lerner, 2001, p. 245).
33. The proposed dimensions are inspired by Warner's account of possible forms that the public and the private can take (2002, p. 29). However, while the categories suggested in this chapter resonate with broader ideas on the meanings of private and public in social life, they are informed by the particular experience of breast cancer patients' use of the Internet.
34. Zerubavel indeed acknowledges the resemblance of his argument to explanations of space as a marker between private and public.
35. www.bcans.org

36. I borrow the concept of a continuum of public and private from Zerubavel (1981, pp. 143–144).
37. The notion of "mobile privatization" was termed by Williams (1974) to characterize a central feature of everyday life in industrial capitalist society, specifically following the move of families from the city to the suburb.
38. The notion of "preserves" in this context is taken from Zerubavel (1981).
39. I do not present the poem in order to secure the interviewee's anonymity.
40. Examples of breast cancer discussion group threads can be found on the forum of www.bcans.org, and Yahoo Breast Cancer Club on www.breastguide.com
41. Examples of breast cancer patients' stories displayed in a table can be found on www.sharedexperience.org and www.breastbiopsy.com/interact_sharestory.jsp
42. I develop this critique elsewhere (see Orgad, 2005b).
43. Beyond the focus on storytelling online in the context of the oral-written and private-public relations, this analysis also calls for a more elaborate consideration of the issue of orality and literacy in relation to online communication more generally. It highlights the need to expand the scope of the discussion beyond synchronous online forums. In existing literature (e.g., Fernback, 2003), the claim for online space as a locus for an oral culture appears restricted to real-time simultaneous online textual environments. Consequently, the kind of online oral culture that Fernback and others depict is derivative of characteristics of synchronous environments, in particular, immediacy and ephemerality. In analyzing patients' online communication, I have insisted on the significance of the oral component of communication also in asynchronous environments, e-mail in particular.
44. In no way do I mean that the feminist "camp" is monolithic in its thinking about the question of public and private. However, it is beyond the scope of this book to inquire into the different approaches to this issue. For the purpose of the current discussion, my intention is to contextualize the arguments made in this chapter about breast cancer online communication and the negotiation of public and private, within the wider discourse on women, Internet use, and the relation between private and public. For recent studies that examine this relation from feminist perspectives, see Youngs (in Harcourt, 1999) and Franklin (2001).
45. There is a crucial U.S./American context to this culture. I develop this issue in the concluding chapter.
46. In making this observation I draw loosely on Gare's discussion of the connection between narrative and agency (2002, p. 97).
47. Bauman cites Alfred Weber.
48. This observation is corroborated by both Sharf's (1997) and Pitts' (2004) studies of breast cancer patients' online communication.
49. Indeed, when reading Ricoeur's seminal volumes on *Time and Narrative* (1984), and later developments of his theory such as the works of Brooks (1994), Gare (2002) and Somers (1994), as well as Giddens' (1991) and Thompson's (1995) accounts of the centrality of narrative in the constitution of agency, it is easy to think of narrating as a key, if not the most fundamental principle, of social agency and human sociality.
50. Clegg Smith draws on the approach of the H Project researchers, which "view public discourse on Computer Mediated Communication as just that: public" (Rafaeli, cited in Sudweeks and Rafaeli, 1995, cited in Clegg Smith, 2004, p. 230).

Bibliography

Acker, K. (1997, January 18). The gift of disease. *The Guardian* (Weekend page), p. T14.

Albom, M. (1998). *Tuesdays with Morrie: An Old Man, A Young Man, and Life's Greatest Lesson*. London: Little, Brown and Company.

Anderson, B., & Tracey, K. (2002). Digital living: The impact (or otherwise) of the Internet on everyday life. In B. Wellman & C. Haythornthwaite (Eds.), *The Internet in Everyday Life* (pp. 45–73). London: Blackwell.

Ang, I. (1985). *Watching Dallas: Soap Opera and the Melodramatic Imagination*. London: Methuen.

Arksey, H. (1998). *RSI and the Experts*. London: UCL Press.

Bakardjieva, M. (2003). Virtual togetherness: An everyday-life perspective. *Media, Culture & Society, 25*(3), 291–313.

Bakardjieva, M., & Smith, R. (2001). The Internet in everyday life: Computer networking from the standpoint of the domestic user. *New Media & Society, 3*(1), 67–83.

Baker, A. (2002). What makes an online relationship successful? Clues from couples who met in cyberspace. *CyberPsychology & Behavior, 5*(4), 363–375.

Bakhtin, M. (1984). *Problems of Dostoevsky's Poetics*. Ed. and trans. C. Emerson. Manchester: Manchester University Press.

Barnes, S. B. (2004). Issues of attribution and identification in online social research. In M. D. Johns, S. S. Chen, & G. J. Hall (Eds.), *Online Social Research: Methods, Issues, & Ethics* (pp. 203–222). New York: Peter Lang.

Barthes, R. (1974). S/Z. London: Blackwell.

———. (1977). *Image-Music-Text: Essays Selected and Translated by Stephen Heath*. London: Fontana.

Bauer, M. W., & Gaskell, G. (Eds.). (2000). *Qualitative Researching with Text, Image and Sound: A Practical Handbook*. London: Sage.

Bauman, Z. (2001, December 29). Quality and inequality. *The Guardian* (Saturday Review), p. 2.

Baym, N. K. (2000). *Tune In, Log On: Soap, Fandom, and Online Community*. London: Sage.

———. (2002). Interpersonal life online. In L. A. Lievrouw & S. Livingstone (Eds.), *Handbook of New Media* (pp. 62–76). London: Sage.

Beck, U. (2001). *Individualization: Institutionalized Individualism and Its Social and Political Consequences*. London: Sage.

Becker, G. (1994). Metaphors in disrupted lives: Infertility and cultural constructions of continuity. *Medical Anthropology Quarterly, 8*(4), 383–410.

Benjamin, W. (1970). *Illuminations*. London: Pimlico.

Berger, A. A. (1997). *Narratives in Popular Culture, Media and Everyday Life*. London: Sage.

Bird, E. S., & Dardenne, R. W. (1988). Myth, chronicle and story: Exploring the narrative qualities of news. In J. W. Carey (Ed.), *Media, Myths, and Narratives: Television and the Press* (pp. 67–86). London: Sage.

Blackman, L. (2004). Self-help, media cultures and the production of female psychopathology. *European Journal of Cultural Studies, 7*(2), 219–236.

Blau, P. M. (1968). Interaction: Social exchange. In D. L. Sills (Ed.), *International Encyclopaedia of the Social Sciences* (Vol. 7). New York: Macmillan and The Free Press.

Boyer, C., Provost, M., & Baujard, V. (2002). *Highlights of the 8th HON Survey of Health and Medical Internet Users*. Health on the Net Foundation. Available at http://www.hon.ch/Survey/8th_HON_results.html (accessed 13 December 2004).

Brooks, P. (1994). *Psychoanalysis and Storytelling*. Oxford: Blackwell.

Bruckman, A. S. (2004). Introduction: Opportunities and challenges in methodology and ethics. In M. D. Johns, S. S. Chen, & G. J. Hall (Eds.), *Online Social Research: Methods, Issues, & Ethics* (pp. 101–104). New York: Peter Lang.

Bruner, J. (1987). Life as narrative. *Social Research, 54*(1), 11–32.

Burrows, R., Nettleton, S., Pleace, N., Loader, B., & Muncer, S. (2000). Virtual community care? Social policy and the emergence of computer mediated social support. *Information, Communication & Society, 3*(1), 95–121.

Bury, M. (1982). Chronic illness as biographical disruption. *Sociology of Health & Illness, 4*(2), 167–182.

———. (1991). The sociology of chronic illness: A review of research and prospects. *Sociology of Health & Illness, 13*(4), 451–468.

———. (2001). Illness narratives: Fact or fiction? *Sociology of Health & Illness, 23*(3), 263–285.

Calman, K. (2001). A study of storytelling, humour and learning in medicine. *Clinical Medicine, 1*(3), 227–229.

Campbell, H. (2003). Congregation and the disembodied: A look at religious community on the Internet. In M. J. P. Wolf (Ed.), *Virtual Morality: Morals, Ethics + New Media*. New York: Peter Lang.

Carlick, A., & Biley, F. C. (2004). Thoughts on the therapeutic use of narrative in the promotion of coping in cancer care. *European Journal of Cancer Care, 13*, 308–317.

Chandler, D. (1998). *Personal Home Pages and the Construction of Identities on the Web*. Available at www.aber.ac.uk/media/Documents/short/webident.html (accessed 13 December 2004).

Charles, C., Whelan, T., Gafni, A., Reyno, L., & Redko, C. (1998). Doing nothing is no choice: Lay constructions of treatment decision-making among women with early-stage breast cancer. *Sociology of Health & Illness, 20*(1), 71–95.

Chen, S. S., Hall, G. J., & Johns, M. D. (2004). Research paparazzi in cyberspace: The voices of the researched. In M. D. Johns, S. S. Chen, & G. J. Hall (Eds.), *Online Social Research: Methods, Issues, & Ethics* (pp. 157–175). New York: Peter Lang.

Clegg Smith, K. M. (2004). Electronic eavesdropping: The ethical issues involved in conducting a virtual ethnography. In M. D. Johns, S. S. Chen, & G. J. Hall (Eds.), *Online Social Research: Methods, Issues, & Ethics* (pp. 223–238). New York: Peter Lang.

Cox, B. (2002). The impact of the Internet on the GP-patient relationship. *Informatics in Primary Care, 10*, 95–98.

Datamonitor. (2002, September 3). *Who is looking for health information online? A segmentation analysis of the online consumer* (Healthcare Report and Services).

Available at www.datamonitor.com/~93f52620bd45498097e7a02e9b9f241c~/healthcare/reports/product_summary.asp?pid=BFHC0470 (accessed 13 December 2004).

DeLillo, D. (2001, December 22). In the ruins of the future. *The Guardian* (Saturday Review), pp. 1–2.

Denzin, N. K. (1999). Cybertalk and the method of instances. In S. Jones (Ed.), *Doing Internet Research: Critical Issues and Methods for Examining the Net* (pp. 107–125). London: Sage.

Dolan, G. (2003). How do patients make use of health-related information from the Internet? Investigating the views of the public and healthcare professionals. *International Journal of Consumer Studies, 27*(3), 241–242.

Donath, J. S. (1999). Identity and deception in the virtual community. In M. Smith & P. Kollock (Eds.), *Communities in Cyberspace* (pp. 29–59). London: Routledge.

Eastin, M. S. (2001). Credibility assessments of online health information: The effects of source expertise and knowledge of content. *Journal of Computer-Mediated Communication, 6*(4). Available at http://www.ascusc.org/jcmc/vol6/issue4/eastin.html (accessed 13 December 2004).

Ehrenreich, B. (2001, December 8). The cult of the pink ribbon. *The Times* (Weekend section), p. 1a.

Ekeh, P. P. (1974). *Social Exchange Theory: The Two Traditions*. London: Heinemann.

Eley, S. (2003, July). *Exploring Online Storytelling and Support Groups*. Paper presented at the fifth seminar of the Virtual Methods Series, Brunel University, U.K. Available at http://www.soc.surrey.ac.uk/virtualmethods/vmpapers/susan.htm (accessed 13 December 2004).

Elgesem, D. (2002). What is special about the ethical issues in online research? *Ethics and Information Technology, 4*(3), 195–203.

Eysenbach, G., Powell, J., Englesakis, M., Rizo, C., & Stern, A. (2004). Health-related virtual communities and electronic support groups: Systematic review of the effects of online peer to peer interactions. *British Medical Journal, 328*, 1166. Available at http://bmj.bmjjournals.com/cgi/content/full/328/7449/1166 (accessed 13 December 2004).

Ferguson, T. (1996). *Health Online*. Reading, MA: Addison-Wesley.

———. (2002). From patients to end users: Quality of online patients networks needs more attention than quality of online health information. *British Medical Journal, 324*, 555–556.

Fernback, J. (2003). Legends on the net: An examination of computer-mediated communication as a locus of oral culture. *New Media & Society, 5*(1), 29–45.

Ferris, B., & Stein, Y. (2002). Care beyond cancer: The culture of creativity. *Illness, Crisis & Loss, 10*(1), 42–50.

Fogel, J. (2002). *Psychological Aspects of Women with Breast Cancer Who Use the Internet*. Unpublished doctoral dissertation, Yeshiva University, New York.

———. (2004). Internet breast health information use and coping among women with breast cancer. *CyberPsychology & Behavior, 7*(1), 59–63.

Fogel, J., Albert, S. M., Schnabel, F., Ditkoff, B. A., & Neugut, A. I. (2002). Internet use and social support in women with breast cancer. *Health Psychology, 21*(4), 398–404.

Fosket, J. (2000). Problematizing biomedicine: Women's constructions of breast cancer knowledge. In L. K. Potts (Ed.), *Ideologies of Breast Cancer: Feminist Perspectives* (pp. 15–36). London: Macmillan Press.

Fox, S. (2003, July 28). *New report on Internet health in the US*. Association of Internet Researchers mailing list. (Available for members from air-e-health@aoir.org).

Frank, A. W. (1995). *The Wounded Storyteller: Body, Illness and Ethics*. Chicago: University of Chicago Press.

Frankenberg, R. (1992). *Time, Health and Medicine*. London: Sage.

Franklin, M. I. (2001). Inside out: Postcolonial subjectivities and everyday life online. *International Feminist Journal of Politics, 3*(3), 387–422.

Friedman, S. S. (1988). Women's autobiographical selves: Theory and practice. In S. Benstock (Ed.), *The Private Self* (pp. 34–62). Chapel Hill: University of North Carolina Press.

Gardiner, M. E. (2000). *Critiques of Everyday Life*. London: Routledge.

Gare, A. (2002). Narratives and culture: The role of stories in self-creation. *Telos, 122*, 80–100.

Giddens, A. (1984). *The Constitution of Society*. Cambridge: Polity Press.

———. (1991). *Modernity and Self Identity: Self and Society in the Late Modern Age*. Cambridge: Polity Press.

Ginossar, T. (2002). *Knowledge Is Power: Health-Information Seeking of Internet Cancer Support Groups Members*. Unpublished doctoral dissertation, University of New Mexico, Albuquerque.

Goffman, E. (1971). *The Presentation of Self in Everyday Life*. London: Penguin.

Goldstein, C. (2003). *Information Overload: Après le Deluge. Ketchum Global Research Network*. Available at http://www.ketchum.com/DisplayWebPage/0,1003,1901,00.html (accessed 13 December 2004).

Grodin, D., & Lindlof, T. R. (1996). *Constructing the Self in a Mediated World*. London: Sage.

Hampton, K., & Wellman, B. (2003). Neighboring in Netville: How the Internet supports community and social capital in a wired suburb. *City and Community, 2*(4), 277–311.

Hardey, M. (1999). Doctor in the house: The Internet as a source of lay health knowledge and the challenge to expertise. *Sociology of Health & Illness, 21*(6), 820–835.

———. (2001). 'E-health': The Internet and the transformation of patients into consumers and producers of health knowledge. *Information, Communication and Society, 4*(3), 388–405.

———. (2002). The story of my illness: Personal accounts of illness on the Internet. *Health, 6*(1), 31–46.

Haythornthwaite, C., & Wellman, B. (2002). The Internet in everyday life: An introduction. In B. Wellman & C. Haythornthwaite (Eds.), *The Internet in Everyday Life* (pp. 3–41). London: Blackwell.

Heiney, S. P. (1995). The healing power of story. *Oncology Nursing Forum, 22*, 899–904.

Herring, S. (1999). Interactional coherence in CMC. *Journal of Computer-Mediated*

Communication, 4(4). Available at http://www.ascusc.org/jcmc/vol4/issue4/herring.html (accessed 13 December 2004).

Hine, C. (2000). *Virtual Ethnography*. London: Sage.

———. (2001). Web pages, authors and audiences: The meaning of a mouse click. *Information, Communication and Society, 4*(2), 182–198.

Hobson, D. (1982). *Crossroads: The Drama of a Soap Opera*. London: Methuen.

Hodgetts, D., & Chamberlain, K. (1999). Medicalization and the depiction of lay people in television health documentary. *Health, 3*(3), 317–333.

Hoffman, L. H., Novak, T. P., & Schlosser, A. E. (2001). The evolution of the digital divide: Examining the relationship of race to Internet access and usage over time. In B. M. Compaine (Ed.), *The Digital Divide: Facing a Crisis or Creating a Myth?* (pp. 47–97). Cambridge, MA: MIT Press.

Houston, T. K., & Allison, J. J. (2002). Users of Internet health information: Differences by health status. *Journal of Medical Internet Research, 4*(2), e7. Available at www.jmir.org/2002/2/e7/index.htm (accessed 13 December 2004).

Hutchby, I. (2001). *Conversation and Technology: From the Telephone to the Internet*. Cambridge: Polity Press.

Hydén, L. C. (1997). Illness and narrative. *Sociology of Health & Illness, 19*(1), 48–69.

Jankowski, N. W., & van Selm, M. (2001, December). *Research Ethics in a Virtual World: Some Guidelines and Illustrations*. Paper presented at the first seminar of the Virtual Methods Series, Royal Holloway, University of London, Egham, Surrey, U.K. Available at http://www.soc.surrey.ac.uk/virtualmethods/vmpapers/nick.htm (accessed 13 December 2004).

Johns, M. D., Chen, S. L. S., & Hall, G. J. (2004). *Online Social Research: Methods, Issues and Ethics*. New York: Peter Lang.

Jones, S. (Ed.). (1998). *Cybersociety 2.0: Revisiting Computer-Mediated Communication and Community*. London: Sage.

———. (2004). Conclusions: Contexting the Network. In P. H. Howard & S. Jones (Eds.), *Society Online: The Internet in Context* (pp. 325–333). London: Sage.

Katz Becker, L. (2000). *Dear Stranger, Dearest Friend*. New York: William Morrow.

King, S. A., & Moreggi, D. (1998). Internet therapy and self-help groups—The pros and cons. In J. Gackenbach (Ed.), *Psychology and the Internet: Intrapersonal, Interpersonal and Transpersonal Implications* (pp. 77–109). San Diego, CA: Academic Press.

Kleinman, A. (1988). *The Illness Narratives: Suffering, Healing and the Human Condition*. New York: Basic Books.

Kollock, P. (1999). The economies of online cooperation: Gifts and public goods in cyberspace. In M. Smith and P. Kollock (Eds.), *Communities in Cyberspace* (pp. 220–239). London: Routledge.

Kozloff, S. (1992). Narrative theory and television. In R. C. Allen (Ed.), *Channels of Discourse, Reassembled* (2nd ed., pp. 67–100). London: Routledge.

Kushner, R. (1977). *Why Me? What Every Woman Should Know About Breast Cancer to Save Her Life*. New York: Henry Holt.

Lambert, H., & Rose, H. (1996) Disembodied knowledge? Making sense of medical science. In A. Irwin & B. Wynne (Eds.), *Misunderstanding Science? The Public Reconstruction of Science and Technology* (pp. 65–83). New York: Cambridge

University Press.

Lasch, U. (1980). *The Culture of Narcissism: American Life in an Age of Diminishing Expectations*. London: Abacus Press.

Lawton, J. (2003). Lay experiences of health and illness: Past research and future agendas. *Sociology of Health & Illness, 25*, 23–40.

Lea, M., & Spears, R. (1995). Love at first byte? In J. Wood & S. Duck (Eds.), *Understudied Relationships: Off the Beaten Track* (pp. 197–240). Thousand Oaks, CA: Sage.

Leopold, E. (1999). *A Darker Ribbon: Breast Cancer, Women, and Their Doctors in the Twentieth Century*. Boston: Beacon Press.

Lerner, B. H. (2001). *The Breast Cancer Wars: Hope, Fear, and the Pursuit of a Cure in Twentieth-Century America*. Oxford: Oxford University Press.

Lévi-Strauss, C. (1968). *Structural Anthropology*. Middlesex: Penguin.

———. (1969). *The Elementary Structures of Kinship*. Boston: Beacon Press.

Lieberman, M. A., & Russo, S. (2002). Self help groups and the Internet: Breast cancer newsgroups. *International Self Help & Self Care, 1*(4), 323–344.

Livingstone, S. (1998). *Making Sense of Television*. London: Routledge.

Livingstone, S., & Lunt, P. (1994). *Talk on Television: Audience Participation and Public Debate*. London: Routledge.

Lorde, A. (1980). *The Cancer Journals*. San Francisco: Spinsters Ink.

Love, S. (2000). *Dr. Susan Love's Breast Book*. Cambridge, MA: Perseus.

Madara, E. J. (1999). From church basements to World Wide Web sites: The growth of self-help support groups online. *Self-Help & Self-Care, 1*(1), 37–48.

Mattingly, C., & Garro, L. C. (Eds.). (2000). *Narrative and the Cultural Construction of Illness and Healing*. Berkeley: University of California Press.

McLellan, F. (1997). A whole other story: The electronic narrative of illness. *Literature and Medicine, 10*(1), 88–107.

Millar, M. S. (1998). *Cracking the Gender Code: Who Rules the Wired World?* Toronto: Second Story Press.

Millard, R. W., & Fintak, P. A. (2002). Use of the Internet by patients with chronic illness. *Disease Management & Health Outcomes, 10*(3), 187–194.

Miller, D., & Slater, D. (2000). *The Internet: An Ethnographic Approach*. London: Berg.

Mitra, A., & Cohen, E. (1999). Analyzing the Web: Distinctions and challenges. In S. Jones (Ed.), *Doing Internet Research: Critical Issues and Methods for Examining the Net* (pp. 179–202). London: Sage.

Murray, J. H. (1998). *Hamlet on the Holodeck: The Future of Narrative in Cyberspace*. Cambridge, MA: MIT Press.

Nie, N. H., & Erbring, L. (2000). *Internet and Society: A Preliminary Report*. Palo Alto, CA: Stanford Institute for the Quantitative Study of Society. Available at http://www.stanford.edu/group/siqss/Press_Release/press_detail.html (accessed 13 December 2004).

Ogden, T. H. (2000). Borges and the art of mourning. *Psychoanalytic Dialogues, 10*(1), 65–88.

Orgad, S. (2004). Just do it! The online communication of breast cancer as a practice of empowerment. In M. Consalvo, N. Baym, J. Hunsinger, K. Jensen, J. Logie, M.

Murero, & L. R. Shade (Eds.), *Internet Research Annual, Vol. 1: Selected Papers from the Association of Internet Researchers Conferences 2000–2002* (pp. 231–240). New York: Peter Lang.

———. (2005a). Moving from online to offline relationships with research participants. In C. Hine (Ed.), *Virtual Methods: Issues in Social Research on the Internet*. Oxford: Berg.

———. (2005b). The political potential of the online communication: The case of breast cancer patients' Internet spaces. *Feminist Media Studies*, *5*(2).

———. (2006). *The Cultural Specificity of Online Communication*. Manuscript submitted for publication.

Paccagnella, L. (1997). Getting the seats of your pants dirty: Strategies for ethnographic research on virtual communities. *Journal of Computer-Mediated Communication*, *3*(1). Available at www.ascusc.org/jcmc/vol3/issue1/paccagnella.html (accessed 13 December 2004).

Peck, J. (1996). The mediated talking cure: Therapeutic framing of autobiography in TV talk shows. In S. Smith & J. Watson (Eds.), *Getting a Life: Everyday Uses of Autobiography* (pp. 134–155). Minneapolis: University of Minnesota Press.

Pew Internet & American Life. (26 November 2000). *The Online Health Care Revolution: How the Web Helps Americans Take Better Care of Themselves*. Available at http://www.pewinternet.org/reports/toc.asp?Report=26 (accessed 13 December 2004).

———. (2002a, May 8). *The Use of the Internet at Major Life Moments*. Available at http://www.pewinternet.org/reports/toc.asp?Report=58 (accessed 13 December 2004).

———. (2002b, May 22). *Vital Decisions: How Internet Users Decide What Information to Trust When They or Their Loved Ones Are Sick*. Available at http://www.pewinternet.org/reports/toc.asp?Report=59 (accessed 13 December 2004).

———. (2003, July 16). *Internet Health Resources: Health Searches and Email Have Become More Commonplace, but There Is Room for Improvement in Searches and Overall Internet Access*. Available at http://www.pewinternet.org/reports/toc.asp?Report=95 (accessed 13 December 2004).

———. (2004, October 10). *Prescription Drugs Online: One in Four American Have Looked Online for Drug Information, but Few Have Ventured into the Online Drug Marketplace*. Available at http://www.pewinternet.org/pdfs/PIP_Prescription_Drugs_Online.pdf (accessed at 13 December 2004).

Pitts, V. (2004). Illness and Internet empowerment: Writing and reading breast cancer in cyberspace. *Health*, *8*(1), 33–59.

Plummer, K. (1990). Herbert Blumer and the life history tradition. *Symbolic Interaction*, *13*(2), 125–145.

Polanyi, L. (1985). *Telling the American Story: A Structural and Cultural Analysis of Conversational Storytelling*. Norwood, NJ: Ablex Publishers.

Polkinghorne, D. E. (1991). Narrative and self-concept. *Journal of Narrative and Life History*, *1*(2&3), 135–151.

Potts, L. K. (2000). Ideologies of Breast Cancer: Feminist Perspectives. London: Macmillan Press.

Preece, J. J., & Ghozati, K. (2001). Experiencing empathy online. In R. E. Rice & J. E.

Katz (Eds.), *The Internet and Health Communication: Experiences and Expectations* (pp. 237–260). London: Sage.

Prior, L. (2003). Belief, knowledge and expertise: The emergence of the lay expert in medical sociology. *Sociology of Health & Illness, 25*, 41–57.

Propp, V. (1968). *Morphology of the Folktale*. Austin: University of Texas Press.

Radley, A. (1993). *Worlds of Illness: Biographical and Cultural Perspectives on Health and Disease*. London: Routledge.

Radway, J. A. (1987). *Reading the Romance: Women, Patriarchy, and Popular Literature*. London: Verso.

Redford, B. (1986). *The Converse of the Pen: Acts of Intimacy in the Eighteenth-Century Familiar Letter*. Chicago: Chicago University Press.

Reents, S. (1999). Impacts of the Internet on the Doctor-Patient Relationship: The Rise of the Internet Health Consumer. *Cyber Dialogue*. Available at www.cyberdialogue.com/pdfs/wp/wp-cch-1999-doctors.pdf (accessed 29 October 2003).

Reeves, P. M. (2000). Coping in cyberspace: The impact of the Internet on the ability of HIV individuals to deal with their illness. *Journal of Health Communication, 5*(1), 47–59.

Rheingold, H. (1994). *The Virtual Community*. London: Secker and Warburg.

Rice, R. E., & Katz, J. E. (Eds.). (2001). *The Internet and Health Communication: Experiences and Expectations*. London: Sage.

Rice, R. E., & Love, G. (1987). Electronic emotion: Socioemotional content in a computer-mediated communication network. *Communication Research, 14*(1), 85–108.

Ricoeur, P. (1980). Narrative time. In W. J. T. Mitchell (Ed.), *On Narrative* (pp. 165–186). Chicago: University of Chicago Press.

———. (1984). *Time and Narrative (Vol. 1)*. Chicago: Chicago University Press.

Rollin, B. (1976). *First, You Cry*. Philadelphia: Lippincott.

Rose, N. (1992). Governing the enterprising self. In P. Heelas & P. Morris (Eds.), *The Values of the Enterprise Culture: The Moral Debate* (pp. 141–164). London: Routledge.

Rosenblum, R. (2000). And till the ghastly tale is told, Sarah Kofman–Primo Levi: Survivors of the Shoah and the dangers of testimony. *European Judaism, 33*(2), 81–103.

Saywell, C., Henderson, L., and Beattie, L. (2000). Sexualized illness: The newsworthy body in media representations of breast cancer. In L. K. Potts (Ed.), *Ideologies of Breast Cancer: Feminist Perspectives* (pp. 37–62). London: Macmillan Press.

Schafer, R. (1980). Narration in the psychoanalytic dialogue. In W. J. T. Mitchell (Ed.), *On Narrative* (pp. 25–49). Chicago: University of Chicago Press.

Seale, C. (2001). Sporting cancer: Struggle language in news reports of people with cancer. *Sociology of Health & Illness, 23*(3), 308–329.

———. (2002). *Media and Health*. London: Sage.

Sennett, R. (1999, April). *Work and Its Narratives*. Plenary talk presented at the British Sociological Association, Glasgow, Scotland.

———. (2001, May). *Theory and Methods in Qualitative Research: Narrative*. A lecture given at the London School of Economics and Political Science. London, U.K.

———. (2002). *DuBois Memorial Lecture*. A lecture given at the London School of Economics and Political Science.

Sharf, B. F. (1997). Communicating breast cancer on-line: Support and empowerment on the Internet. *Women & Health, 26*(1), 65–84.

Shaw, B. R. (2000). *The Functions and Influence of Insightful Disclosure within Computer-Mediated Support Groups on Women with Breast Cancer*. Unpublished doctoral dissertation, University of Wisconsin, Madison.

Shaw, B. R., McTavish, F., Hawkins, R., Gustafson, D. H., & Pingree, S. (2000). Experiences of women with breast cancer: Exchanging social support over the CHESS computer network. *Journal of Health Communication, 5*(2), 135–159.

Silverstone, R. (1983). The right to speak: On a poetic for television documentary. *Media, Culture & Society, 5*, 137–154.

———. (1984). A structure for a modern myth: Television and the transsexual. *Semiotica, 49*(1–2), 95–138.

———. (1988). Television, myth and culture. In J. W. Carey (Ed.), *Media, Myths, and Narratives: Television and the Press* (pp. 20–44). London: Sage.

———. (1994). *Television and Everyday Life*. London: Routledge.

———. (1999). *Why Study the Media?* London: Sage.

Slater, D. (2002). Social relationships and identity online and offline. In L. Lievrouw & S. Livingstone (Eds.), *The Handbook of New Media* (pp. 534–547). London: Sage.

Somers, M. R. (1994). The narrative constitution of identity: A relational and network approach. *Theory and Society, 23*, 605–649.

Sontag, S. (1978). Illness as Metaphor. New York: Vintage Books.

Spence, D. P. (1982). *Narrative Truth and Historical Truth: Meaning and Interpretation in Psychoanalysis*. New York: W. W. Norton.

Stacey, J. (1997). *Teratologies: A Cultural Study of Cancer*. London: Routledge.

Stacey, M. (1988). *The Sociology of Health and Healing*. London: Routledge.

Stone, A. R. (1995). *The War of Desire and Technology at the Close of the Mechanical Age*. Cambridge, MA: MIT Press.

Sundén, J. (2003). *Material Virtualities: Approaching Online Textual Embodiment*. New York: Peter Lang.

Szymborska, W. (1993). *Miracle Fair: Selected Poems of Wislawa Szymborska*. New York: Norton.

Tabbi, J. (2000). Narrative. In T. Swiss (Ed.), *Unspun: Key Concepts for Understanding the World Wide Web* (pp. 138–147). New York: New York University Press.

Terry, J., & Calvert, M. (Eds.). (1997). *Processed Lives: Gender and Technology in Everyday Life*. London: Routledge.

Thompson, J. B. (1995). *The Media and Modernity: A Social Theory of the Media*. Cambridge: Polity Press.

Turkle, S. (1996). *Life on the Screen: Identity in the Age of the Internet*. London: Weidenfeld & Nicolson.

Turner, V. (1969). *The Ritual Process: Structures and Anti-Structures*. Ithaca, NY: Cornell University Press.

van Gennep, A. (1960). *The Rites of Passage*. London: Routledge & Kegan Paul.

Walker, K. (2000). "It's difficult to hide it": The presentation of self on Internet home pages. *Qualitative Sociology*, *32*(1), 99–120.

Walstrom, M. K. (1999). *'Starvation...Is Who I Am': From Eating Disorder to Recovering Identities Through Narrative Co-Construction in an Internet Support Group*. Unpublished doctorial dissertation, University of Illinois at Urbana-Champaign.

Warner, M. (2002). *Publics and Counterpublics*. New York: Zen Books.

Webb, S. (2001). Avatar culture: Narrative, power and identity in virtual world environments. *Information, Communication & Society*, *4*(4), 560–594.

Wellman, B. (1999). The network community. In B. Wellman (Ed.), *Networks in the Global Village* (pp. 1–48). Boulder, CO: Westview.

White, H. (1980). The value of narrativity in the representation of reality. In W. J. T. Mitchell (Ed.), *On Narrative* (pp. 1–23). Chicago: University of Chicago Press.

White, M. (1992). *Tele-Advising: Therapeutic Discourse in American Television*. Chapel Hill: University of North Carolina Press.

Whitten, P. (Ed.). (2001). Health and the new media. *Journal of Computer-Mediated Communications*, *6*(4), Special Issue.

Williams, G. (1984). The genesis of chronic illness: Narrative reconstruction. *Sociology of Health & Illness*, *6*, 175–200.

Williams, R. (1974). *Television: Technology and Cultural Form*. London: Fontana.

Wynn, E., & Katz, J. E. (1997). Hyperbole over cyberspace: Self-presentation and social boundaries in Internet home pages and discourse. *Information Society*, *13*, 297–327.

Yalom, I. D. (1970). *The Theory and Practice of Group Psychotherapy*. London: Basic Books.

Yaphe, J., Rigge, M., Herxheimer, A., McPherson, A., Miller, R., Shepperd, S., & Ziebland, S. (2000). The use of patients' stories by self-help groups: A survey of voluntary organizations in the UK on the register of the College of Health. *Health Expectations*, *3*, 176–181.

Youngs, G. (1999). Virtual voices: Real lives. In W. Harcourt (Ed.), *Women@internet: Creating New Cultures in Cyberspace* (pp. 55–68). London: Zed Books.

Zerubavel, E. (1981). *Hidden Rhythms: Schedules and Calendars in Social Life*. Chicago: University of Chicago Press.

Index

N

O

P

R

S

Z

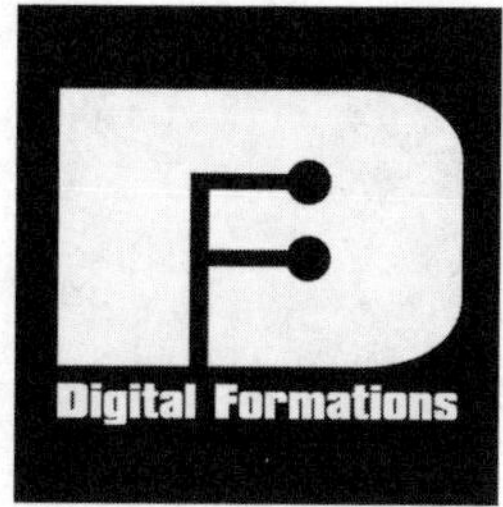

General Editor: *Steve Jones*

Digital Formations is an essential source for critical, high-quality books on digital technologies and modern life. Volumes in the series break new ground by emphasizing multiple methodological and theoretical approaches to deeply probe the formation and reformation of lived experience as it is refracted through digital interaction. **Digital Formations** pushes forward our understanding of the intersections—and corresponding implications—between the digital technologies and everyday life. The series emphasizes critical studies in the context of emergent and existing digital technologies.

Other recent titles include:

Leslie Shade
Gender and Community in the Social Construction of the Internet

John T. Waisanen
Thinking Geometrically

Mia Consalvo & Susanna Paasonen
Women and Everyday Uses of the Internet

Dennis Waskul
Self-Games and Body-Play

David Myers
The Nature of Computer Games

Robert Hassan
The Chronoscopic Society

M. Johns, S. Chen, & G. Hall
Online Social Research

C. Kaha Waite
Mediation and the Communication Matrix

Jenny Sunden
Material Virtualities

Helen Nissenbaum & Monroe Price
Academy and the Internet

To order other books in this series please contact our Customer Service Department:

(800) 770-LANG (within the US)
(212) 647-7706 (outside the US)
(212) 647-7707 FAX

To find out more about the series or browse a full list of titles, please visit our website:

WWW.PETERLANGUSA.COM